CONTENTS

Note on cross-references to SCIENTIFIC AMERICAN *articles:* Articles included in this book are referred to by chapter number and title; articles not included in this book but available as Offprints are referred to by title, date of publication and Offprint number; articles not in this book and not available as Offprints are referred to by title and date of publication.

Immunology

Recognition and Response

. . .

READINGS FROM
SCIENTIFIC AMERICAN MAGAZINE

Edited by

William E. Paul

National Institute of Allergy and Infectious Diseases

W. H. FREEMAN AND COMPANY
New York

Some of the SCIENTIFIC AMERICAN articles in *Immunology: Recognition and Response* are available as separate Offprints. For a complete list of articles now available as Offprints, write to Product Manager, Marketing Department, W. H. Freeman and Company, 41 Madison Avenue, New York, NY 10010.

Library of Congress Cataloging-in-Publication Data

Immunology : recognition and response : readings from Scientific American magazine / edited by William E. Paul.
    p.   cm.
   Articles published 1980–1990.
   Includes bibliographic references and index.
   ISBN 0-7167-2223-2 : $11.95
   1. Immune response. I. Paul, William E. II. Scientific American.
QR186.I4684   1991
616.07′9 — dc20   90-22980
                          CIP

Printed in the United States of America

1 2 3 4 5 6 7 8 9 0 RRD 9 9 8 7 6 5 4 3 2 1 0

Cover Image: Artwork featuring different types of white blood cells that comprise the orchestra of the human immune system, the body's defense mechanism. The maturation of cells derived from bone marrow is featured at bottom left. There are three main types of white cells — lymphocytes, leucocytes and monocytes (the large macrophage at top right is a monocyte). Lymphocytes originate in the bone marrow and mature there or in the thymus — hence the names *B* lymphocytes (blue, center right) and *T* lymphocytes (orange, bottom). *B* cells produce antibodies, chemicals that disable invading microorganisms. Some *T* cells attack other cells infected with viruses directly.

Preface

The immune system of vertebrates provides a remarkable defense against infectious agents that has allowed humans and other higher organisms to flourish in the midst of an environment replete with potentially pathogenic microorganisms. This protective role of the immune system was implicit in the use of vaccination with the cowpox virus (vaccinia) to protect against the often fatal infection with the closely related smallpox virus (variola). Indeed, it is one of the greatest triumphs of medicine that smallpox, once among the leading causes of death throughout the world, has been entirely eliminated from the earth through an aggressive program of vaccination.

Immunology as a science may be regarded as having begun barely a century ago with the remarkable demonstration by Louis Pasteur that injection of an attenuated form of the chicken cholera bacillus protected birds against what would have been a lethal innoculum of the intact organism. This work was rapidly followed by a series of brilliant experiments by Pasteur, Heinrich Koch, Emil A. von Behring, Paul Ehrlich and others that established many of the key features of the immune response, including its inducibility and specificity. In many respects, the period immediately following Pasteur's initial findings constituted a scientific revolution as profound and exciting as the one that is now transforming biology.

Not only does the immune system have the potential to provide us with induced protection against infectious agents, it is central to our survival. This critical role of a functioning immune system to normal life is tragically illustrated by the inability of individuals with major deficiencies in this system, such as children with severe combined immunodeficiency disease or patients with AIDS, to survive without extraordinary measures. Even partial deficiencies of the immune system, such as the agammaglobulinemias (disorders in which antibodies are not made), open patients to severe and recurrent infections unless they are appropriately treated.

The immune system mediates its protective function through its ability to recognize virtually any foreign molecule and to make a response that involves an enormous amplification of the recognition elements and the engagement of potent effector mechanisms that either eliminate or neutralize the pathogenic agent. Thus, as illustrated by the subtitle of this volume, recognition and response are two of the hallmarks of the immune response.

The articles chosen for inclusion in this volume illustrate many of the key facets of the system. Section I is a discussion of the theoretical basis of modern immunology, the clonal-selection theory, whose introduction in 1959 had a profound effect on the field. Section II discusses in detail the cellular and molecular basis of immunological specificity, including the means through which the immune system is able to recognize virtually any foreign macromolecule, but can "tolerate" the presence of comparable materials that are produced by the individual. Section III considers the means through which the immune system regulates its function and the nature of one of its most potent effector mechanisms. Thus, it involves a discussion of the molecular mediators of immunity, agents produced by cells of the immune system that act on other components of the system, often at picomolar concentrations. It further discusses the remarkable capacity of a subset of immune cells to destroy other cells that bear antigens for which the killer cells are specific. Section IV consists of two chapters that deal with the importance of the immune system in the clinical arena, including the consequences of the failure of immunological tolerance and the consequent effects of immunity directed against tissues of the host, as well as the clinical potential of enhancing immunity through the use of endogenous products of the immune system. Section V is devoted to one of the most remarkable advances of immunology, the monoclonal antibody technique and some potential uses of these antibodies, such as the catalysis of chemical reactions and the targeting of specific cells and tissues, most particularly cancer cells, for destruction by potent toxic agents that can be linked to such antibodies.

These chapters provide a striking picture of modern immunology and should allow an understanding of both the basic principles of the immune system, of its participation in initiation and development of a variety of diseases, and of how it may be manipulated to enhance its protective capacity.

William E. Paul

CLONAL SELECTION
The Central Paradigm of Immunology

...

Introduction

In the immune system's need to have a recognition system of sufficient breadth to deal with the vast and changing array of structures displayed on potentially pathogenic microbes, it is faced with the problem of developing a molecular repertoire large enough to react with the universe of foreign structures (antigens) while also finding a way to exempt from attack structures on its own tissues. The cellular and molecular basis of repertoire acquisition and of immunological tolerance (the failure to respond to self-antigens) constitute two of the key and biologically most unique challenges that face the immune system.

As discussed in Chapter 1, "The Clonal Selection Theory," by Gordon L. Ada and Sir Gustav Nossal, the immune response represents an evolved system that allows these twin goals to be met with a high degree of reliability. Rather than endowing all the specific cells of the immune system (the lymphocytes) with the capacity to recognize the full range of foreign antigens, the system has developed a strategy in which each individual cell displays a single set of essentially identical recognition structures (receptors) on its surface. The combining specificity of these receptors is different for each lymphocyte. Thus, the challenge of recognizing a universe of foreign structures is met by the development of an internal universe of lymphocytes, each bearing distinct receptors of differing specificity. When an infectious agent enters the body, the various antigens that it displays are recognized by the specific cells of the immune system that bear receptors complementary to those antigens. This recognition leads to a selective proliferation by the specific lymphocytes, resulting in the development of a clone of cells with essentially identical receptors. The twin properties of cellular selection and clonal expansion led to the name of the theory that constitutes the central paradigm of the immune system — the clonal-selection theory. Clonal selection allows the development of an enormous repertoire by the "simple" expedient of using the equivalent of a genetic random structure generator in individual precursors of immunocompetent cells to generate lymphocytes capable of recognizing virtually any antigenic substance and provides for immunological tolerance by the elimination or inactivation of those lymphocytes that bear receptors capable of recognizing self-antigens.

The simultaneous proposal of this theory by F. Macfarlane Burnet in Melbourne and David W. Talmage in Denver marks the beginning of modern immunology. Virtually all aspects of modern immunological science are based on the underpinnings provided by the insight of these two remarkable scientists.

The Clonal-Selection Theory

*The antibodies that defend the body from foreign invasion are
remarkably diverse. It took nearly 100 years to define and
substantiate a theory that could account for their formation.*

. . .

Gordon L. Ada and Sir Gustav Nossal
August, 1987

How do cells make antibodies in such enormous variety? Today that question has largely been answered, and the protective proteins produced by the immune system are the servants of medicine and research. Not so long ago, however, antibodies were much more mysterious. Their origin and mode of action were the focus of several competing and conflicting theories.

Antibody formation is problematic because of the almost incredible diversity of antigens, the foreign substances that provoke an immune response. One antibody can neutralize just one type of antigen — but antigens come in a variety of shapes, sizes and chemical compositions. Bacteria and their toxins, viruses, pollen grains, incompatible blood cells and man-made molecules can all act as antigens. To catch each type of intruder, the white blood cells called B lymphocytes must create hoards of customized antibodies.

How antigens guide the immune reaction was the chief point of contention among early theorists, splitting them into two camps. One school of thought held that antigens serve as templates that direct the design of matching antibodies. The other school believed lymphocytes maintain a pool of predesigned antibodies from which an antigen selects its closest match. In the past 30 years the combined efforts of many investigators in many countries have clarified the biological basis of immunity and resolved the conflict. The second viewpoint has triumphed, in a doctrine called the clonal-selection theory of antibody formation.

This chapter documents the creation and validation of the clonal-selection theory. The theory was proposed in essence almost 100 years ago, but it then fell into and out of favor with the vicissitudes of evidence and speculation. Both of us were privileged to take part in the research that brought the theory into its own in the 1960s's.

The search for the mechanism of antibody formation began late in the 19th century, by which time Louis Pasteur's germ theory of disease had become generally accepted. Several groups began to study the reaction between bacterial toxins and the "antitoxins" that appear after infection in the blood serum, the fluid component of blood. The German bacteriologist Emil A. von Behring called the substances Antikörper, or antibodies.

Reactions between antibodies and antigens could be observed in a test tube because the reactants formed aggregates visible to the unaided eye. It soon became apparent that bacterial products were not the only thing that could spur antibody production. Other natural substances such as the proteins in milk and "foreign" cells could also engage the immune response of the "host" animal.

In 1890 von Behring, who had developed an antitoxin against diphtheria, met another German medical scientist, Paul Ehrlich (see Figure 1.1). Ehrlich later published a landmark paper describing a technique for measuring diphtheria antibodies in preparations like von Behring's. The technique allowed such preparations to be standardized and consequently made diphtheria antiserum safe for clinical practice.

In devising his technique for measuring antibodies Ehrlich established the basis for a quantitative approach to immunology. The new, quantitative observations revealed the immune response to be an explosive proliferation of antibodies following contact with an infectious agent. To explain how foreign substances could induce this reaction, Ehrlich developed his side-chain theory of antibody formation (see Figure 1.2).

Announced at the turn of the century, the side-chain theory postulated that a white blood cell's surface bore receptors with side chains to which foreign substances became chemically linked. This binding prompted the cell to produce copies of the bound receptor in great excess. The superfluous receptors — antibodies — were shed into the blood. Ehrlich's critical assumption was that cells naturally made side chains that were capable of binding all foreign substances.

Some critics of Ehrlich's theory opposed the idea of a chemical union between the antigen and its receptor. Other workers accepted the concept but debated the mechanism of antigen binding. Did the cell "swallow" the antigen-receptor complex, or was the reaction reversible, with receptors clutching antigens and then letting go? Amidst these disputes the study of antigen-antibody reactions and antibody specificity took on greater importance. It was known that antibodies begin circulating in the blood of an animal soon after its first contact with an antigen and that a second contact with the same antigen results in a more rapid and more potent response. No one knew, however, just how particular these antibodies are.

FORGING THE TEMPLATE THEORY

Many investigators approached the question of antibody specificity by examining the effects of modified antigens. In 1906 Ernest P. Pick and Friedrich P. Obermayer in Germany showed that attaching chemical groups such as iodine or nitrate to a protein profoundly changes its antigenic properties. At about the same time the Austrian-born immunologist Karl Landsteiner began pursuing a similar experimental strategy. His work, most of which was done at the Rockefeller Institute for Medical Research, would span three decades and demonstrate conclusively the exquisite specificity of antibodies.

Landsteiner coupled antigenic proteins with a great variety of chemical groups, some of which came from pathogenic microbes and some of which were synthesized in a test tube. Each altered molecule evoked a different antibody. Landsteiner thereby confirmed Pick and Obermeyer's evidence that chemical subunits of a larger antigenic structure could determine immunological specificity. These determinants, which were simply foreign molecular patterns, did not themselves constitute antigens: they could not initiate antibody production or form aggregates with antibodies unless they were linked to a carrier molecule.

It is now evident that many determinants cannot generate an immunological response on their own because they are too small; they need to be attached to a larger molecule in order to be recognized. Eighty years ago, however, the finding that determinants were not antigens was rather puzzling. Furthermore, the discovery of antigenic determinants indicated that the diversity of foreign substances confronting the immune system was much greater than had been suspected. It was now clear that a single intruder, such as a bacterium, could bear thousands of determinants and initiate the production of thousands of different antibodies.

From Landsteiner's studies it became apparent that an animal could manufacture a practically unlimited range of antibodies and that it could even make antibodies against novel artificial compounds. These discoveries invited the conclusion that a host animal could not inherently possess the information it uses in responding to such a wide spectrum of antigens. Ehrlich's side-chain theory was therefore discarded in favor of the concept that antigens can somehow direct antibody specificity as the antibodies are synthesized in the blood cell.

Figure 1.1 CONCEPTUAL FATHER of the clonal-selection theory, German physician Paul Ehrlich, proposed in 1900 that antibodies exist as specific receptors on cell surfaces. The Nobel laureate also helped to develop an antiserum for the treatment of diphtheria and later formulated a drug for syphilis.

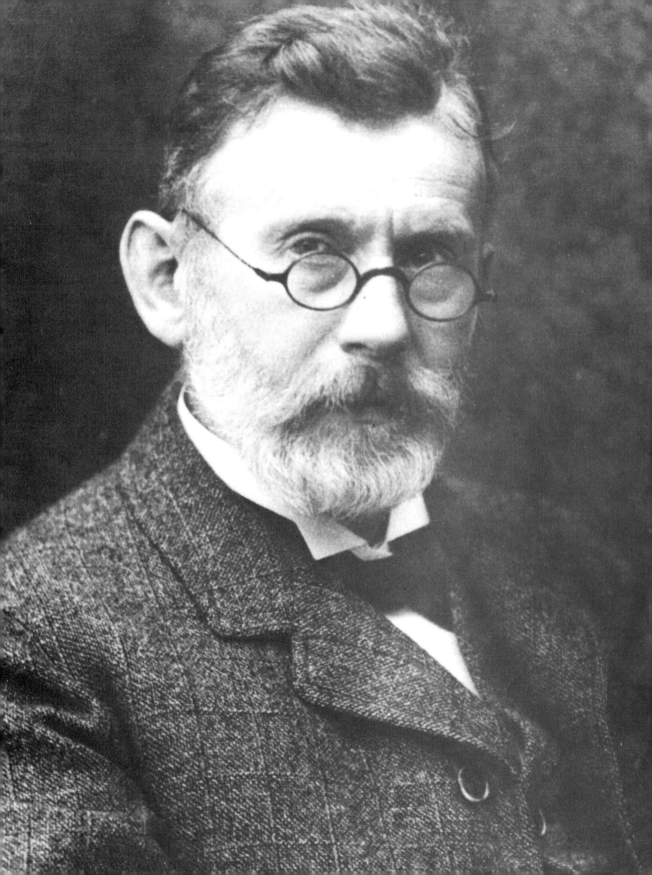

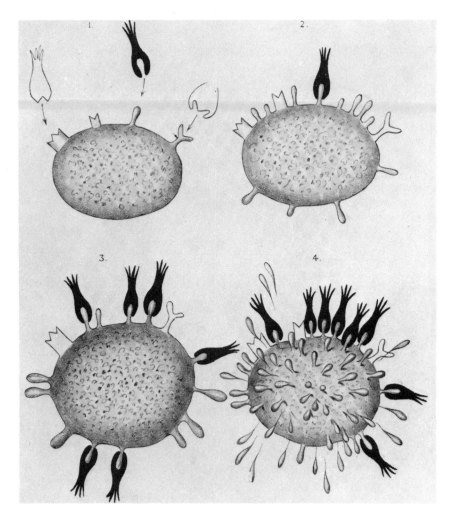

Figure 1.2 EHRLICH'S ILLUSTRATION of the side-chain theory accompanied the 1900 paper in which he announced his new idea. Here a foreign substance (*black*) binds to a cell receptor (*1, 2*), stimulating the cell to make and release identical receptors—antibodies (*3, 4*).

How could an antigen mold the conformation of an antibody? In the early 1930's a number of proposals were advanced, all of them necessarily conjectural. Friedrich Breinl and Felix Haurowitz of the University of Prague and Stuart Mudd and Jerome Alexander of the University of Pennsylvania thought antibodies were manufactured in direct contact with their antigens, adopting a shape and a chemical affinity that were complementary to those of the antigen. They suggested that antibodies molded by different antigens might differ in their protein composition; that is, the sequences of amino acid building blocks making up the antibodies might differ. Others, most notably Linus Pauling, contended that a wide variety of binding specificities could result merely from folding the same antibody protein in different ways. Again, the folding would be guided by the antigen template. Collectively these suppositions were called the template theory of antigen formation. The theory held sway for a quarter of a century.

These arguments about mechanisms of antibody formation took place before the dawn of molecular biology in the 1950's; they were based more on concepts than on experimental data. Hence the first serious challenge to the template theory came from biologists, not biochemists. Three scientists as remarkable as any who had preceded them marshaled the incriminating evidence. Two would later receive Nobel prizes, as had von Behring, Ehrlich and Landsteiner before them.

A CRACK IN THE TEMPLATE

The first comprehensive attack was launched in 1955 by the Danish immunologist Niels Kaj Jerne. In a paper published that year, Jerne recalled that in 1949 two Australian investigators, F. Macfarlane Burnet and Frank J. Fenner, had noted several observations the template theory could not accommodate. First, the theory could not explain the apparently exponential rise in antibody production during the early stages of an immune response. If an antigenic template was required to make each antibody, it was hard to envision how antibodies could so quickly outnumber their templates. Moreover, the theory could not account for the boost in antibody production that occurs when an animal encounters a given antigen for the second time. Why should reintroducing a template give rise to more copies of antibody than the initial contact did?

The fact that antibody production continues long after the antigen is gone also posed problems for the template theory, since it was thought antibody-producing cells were short-lived. Furthermore, the template theory made no provision for the fact that, as the immune reaction progressed, antibodies seemed to become better at binding their target antigens.

Perhaps the most compelling challenge Burnet and Fenner had noted was the phenomenon of immunological tolerance. Tolerance, the failure to launch an immunological campaign against a given antigen, had been recognized not long before Burnet and Fenner published their criticisms. Tolerance keeps an animal from making antibodies against itself and can be acquired for foreign antigens, if the antigens are administered before or at birth. In contrast to immunity, tolerance cannot be maintained unless the antigen persists in the animal. On the subject of immunological tolerance the template theory was silent.

In his article "The Natural-Selection Theory of Antibody Formation" Jerne drew on these criticisms to formulate a notion that would have sounded familiar to Ehrlich, namely that any given animal possesses small numbers of antibodies against all antigens. An immune response occurs when an antigen binds to an antibody and the antigen-antibody complex interacts with white blood cells, stimulating the production and release of the same specific antibody in great quantities. Jerne's proposal was supported by the observation that normal blood serum always contains globulins, nonspecific antibody proteins that at the time seemed to differ from antibodies only in their lack of specificity. Jerne also cited a review by Robert Doerr of the University of Basel that summarized the evidence for "natural" antibodies — antibodies generated without an antigenic stimulus.

At the University of Colorado's School of Medicine at Denver, David W. Talmage read Jerne's proposal and saw the similarities between Jerne's thinking and Ehrlich's side-chain theory. Talmage went a bit further. In a 1957 paper he suggested that replicating cells as well as freely circulating antibody molecules must be a central feature of the immune response. Cells are selected for multiplication, he contended, when the antibody they synthesize matches the invading antigen. Talmage also pointed out that a cancerous antibody-producing cell gives rise to a remarkably homogeneous flood of antibodies, indicating that individual cells might "specialize" in producing a particular antibody.

In retrospect it is obvious that Jerne and Talmage had laid the foundations for the clonal-selection theory of antibody formation in their two papers. It remained for Burnet, however, to draw together the new conceptualizations that his musings with Fenner had sparked. Burnet had been struggling to define a mechanism whereby an antigen's contact with a cell would trigger a self-replicating system. He first envisioned antigens as instructors for adaptive enzymes that, having taken the measure of the antigen once, could then proceed with antibody synthesis in the antigen's absence. Later he proposed that antigens interact directly with the genetic material of a cell. These models did not survive, but they did lead him to stress the importance of cellular function and replication in antibody production.

CLONAL SELECTION

For Burnet, Jerne's article supplied the missing link: the notion that the body is endowed with preexisting antibodies to recognize all antigens. Echoing Ehrlich and Talmage, he proposed that the binding of an antigen with an antibody-cum-receptor triggers the cell to multiply and manufacture more of the same receptor. Then Burnet went out on a conceptual limb: he asserted that each cell and its clones, or offspring, can produce just one kind of receptor. He coined the term "clonal selection" to describe his theory (see Figure 1.3).

The clonal-selection theory was attractive to Burnet because it answered several of his earlier criticisms of the template theory. The exponential rise in antibody production following contact with an antigen results from the exponential rise in the number of antibody-producing cells. The secondary reaction to an antigen is more potent and rapid than the first because there are more cells to respond after the initial antigenic stimulation. Once an entire cadre of cells making a particular antibody has been generated, prolonged exposure to the antigen is not necessary to maintain antibody production. The binding ability of the antibodies improves with time because the antigen "selects" for replication cells carrying genetic mutations that promote the match between antibody and antigen. Finally, the clonal-

selection theory explained immunological tolerance as the deletion of an entire clone of cells, which could occur before or soon after birth or later, if an antigen overwhelmed the metabolic capabilities of the cells.

Burnet conceived of the immune response as a kind of Darwinian microcosm. The antibody-producing cells, like any organism in an ecosystem, are subject to mutation and selection; the fittest survive —fitness being literally, in this case, the "fit" between a cell's antibody and the antigen. In 1957, after seeing Talmage's review, Burnet submitted his manuscript to an obscure journal. He may have been conscious of the flaws in his earlier proposals; it was not until 1958 that he began writing a book to elaborate on his theory, and it was even later that he published his evolving views in more prominent journals.

Burnet developed and aggressively promoted the clonal-selection theory over the next decade. The

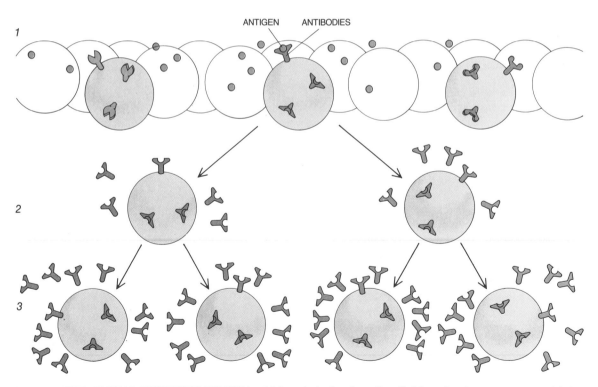

Figure 1.3 THE CLONAL-SELECTION THEORY, which gained favor in the 1960's, holds that antibody-producing cells have specific receptors and that each cell makes just one kind. If an antigen matches a receptor, it binds (1), inducing the cell to divide and make more receptors (2). As in Ehrlich's model, the receptors, or antibodies, are shed from the cell surface into the blood (3).

1960 Nobel prize he and P. B. Medawar shared acknowledged his conceptual accomplishments in understanding acquired immunological tolerance, but Burnet himself believed articulating and promoting the clonal-selection theory was his more significant achievement. In 1984 Jerne would also receive a Nobel Prize for his theoretical contributions to immunology, the most fundamental of which was his role in developing the selective theory.

In February, 1957, one of us (Nossal) had started a research fellowship in Burnet's laboratory to examine the problems of immunological tolerance in fetal mice. When Burnet announced the clonal-selection theory later that year, it seemed natural to suggest, in Popperian style, an experiment that would refute it.

ONE CELL, ONE ANTIBODY?

Like every student of Burnet's, Nossal was encouraged to read the current literature on viruses. He became intrigued by reports that the cells used for growing animal viruses could be isolated and kept alive in single-cell cultures. The experimental design lent itself to testing of the clonal-selection theory. Central to Burnet's thinking was the tenet that one cell produced just one kind of antibody. If a single antibody-producing cell could be isolated, it might be possible to determine whether that cell was making more than one kind of antibody.

By a fortunate coincidence Joshua Lederberg, then at the University of Wisconsin at Madison, also happened to be spending a few months in Burnet's laboratory on a Fulbright fellowship. Lederberg, one of the fathers of bacterial genetics, had considerable experience in capturing individual bacterial cells in tiny droplets of nutrient broth for study under the light microscope. Lederberg volunteered his skills for the experiment; the investigators planned to use bacterial motion as the indicator of antibody production (see Figure 1.4).

It was known that bacteria could be stopped dead in their tracks by antibodies against flagella, the delicate, hairlike structures that propel the microbes. Nossal and Lederberg immunized rats with two different flagellar antigens; a few days later they removed the rats' lymph nodes — structures that, along with the spleen, are a major site of antibody production.

The group teased the tissue apart with fine needles to create a suspension of single cells and introduced the cells one by one into droplets no larger than a millionth of a milliliter. A layer of mineral oil surrounded the droplets to keep them from evaporating. After a brief incubation five to 10 rapidly swimming bacteria with identical flagella were added to each droplet and observed under a microscope. If the bacteria were immobilized, indicating the presence of one type of antibody, the workers inserted bacteria that had the other kind of flagella.

The investigators found that whereas many cells made antibodies against one type of flagella, no cell made antibodies against both types. Thus the one-cell, one-antibody rule was established by an experiment designed to disprove it.

DISARMING CROSS-REACTIONS

In 1959 Nossal joined Lederberg at the Stanford University School of Medicine to set up a new laboratory of immunology. There he entered into a two-year collaboration with Olavi Mäkelä of the University of Helsinki that confirmed and extended the conclusions of Burnet's group. The collaboration fired Mäkelä's imagination, and on returning to Helsinki he turned his attention to immunological cross-reaction, a phenomenon in which antibodies raised against one antigen react against other, similar antigens. He decided to use single-cell cultures for his investigations.

Mäkelä provoked antibody formation with bacterial viruses called phages. He quantified a cell's antibody response by measuring how many phages each cell could disarm, or render unable to infect their host bacteria. Before testing antibodies from single cells, he examined the pool of antibodies in the blood serum of an immunized animal. There he found what the textbooks had taught him to expect: animals immunized with an immunogenic phage A develop antibodies that neutralize phage A very well but that cross-react with phage B with an efficiency of only 20 percent.

When Mäkelä looked at the antibodies in single-cell droplets, his results were quite different. The antibodies of each cell had a different degree of specificity for phage A. Most neutralized phage A better than phage B — but not all. Each cell seemed to be making antibodies with slightly different properties. The reactions Mäkelä had observed in the serum simply reflected the cumulative effect of many idiosyncratic cells, each one "doing its own thing." That discovery was exactly what the clonal-selection theory predicted.

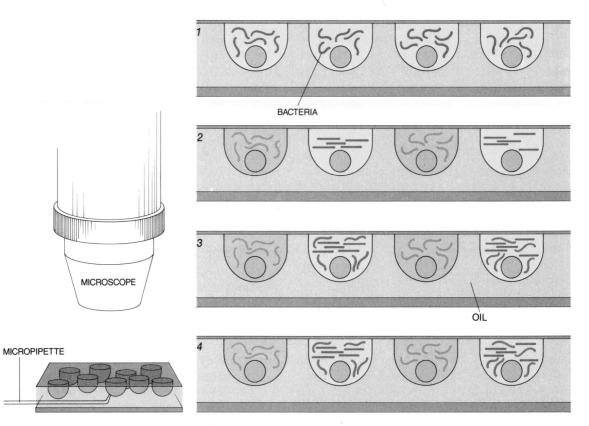

Figure 1.4 SINGLE-CELL CULTURES enabled immunologists to test how many different antibodies one cell could produce. Rats were immunized against two motile bacteria (*red, green*); their lymph-node cells were isolated in drops of nutrient medium, where they could be viewed with a microscope (*left*). Bacteria were added to the drops with a micropipette (*1*). If a cell immobilized one kind of bacterium (*2*), the second kind was injected (*3*). Many cells could stop either kind of bacterium; none stopped both kinds (*4*).

THE TEMPLATE THEORY FALLS

For almost five years after Nossal's experiments the study of antibody formation by single cells was virtually the private preserve of Nossal, Mäkelä and those they had trained. Then, in 1963, Jerne and Albert A. Nordin of the University of Pittsburgh developed a much simpler method for detecting the presence of antibodies secreted by single cells. The spleen and lymph-node cells of mice immunized with sheep red blood cells are spread on a gelatin plate coated with the blood cells. When certain proteins are added, a clear zone appears around each cell producing antibodies. The technique is flexible and is particularly accurate for counting active cells. Its availability led many more laboratories to study the questions raised by Burnet's theory.

While other investigators explored the predictions of the clonal-selection theory, we began our five-year collaboration in 1962 with an experiment we hoped would resolve once and for all the viability of the template theory. We wanted to trace the path of antigen molecules in the body. By this time it was clear that antibodies and all other proteins are manufactured by specialized structures called polyribosomes. If the template theory was correct, each polyribosome would have to be associated with an antigen molecule or at least a substantial fragment of one. Each cell contains thousands of active polyribosomes; it stood to reason that each antibody-producing cell would have to contain many copies of the antigen or its fragments.

The antigens of bacterial flagella served as our tools once again. We attached a radioactive form of iodine to a flagellar antigen so that we could locate the antigen and its "labeled" fragments by looking for radioactivity in cells or tissue samples from the injected animal. Not a single antibody-producing cell contained a detectable quantity of the "hot" antigen, even though our methods were sensitive enough to find 10 antigen molecules per cell. Instead we discovered most of the antigen in a kind of scavenger cell known as a macrophage. This evidence was quite inconsistent with the predictions of the template theory.

In spite of our extensive use of hot antigens in tracking immunologically active cells, it did not occur to us to check for antibodies in unimmunized animals. Yet one of the most controversial claims of the clonal-selection theory was that a small number of natural receptors (antibodies) for all antigens are present prior to immunization. It could have been contended that the number is so small that the receptors can easily escape detection, with the result that some globulins in the blood serum appear to be nonspecific.

Two investigators from the Hebrew University of Jerusalem reasoned that the signal from radioactive antigens bound to the receptors might be strong enough to be detected. David Naor and Dov Sulitzeanu exposed the spleen cells of unimmunized mice to a labeled antigen and looked for evidence that the antigen had bound. They were assuming, in accordance with the clonal-selection theory, that a small number of cells would have receptors reactive with the antigen. Hence they expected to find traces of radioactivity on a very few cells.

That is exactly what Naor and Sulitzeanu found. Moreover, as the clonal-selection theory predicted, immunized animals yielded more antigen-binding cells than unimmunized animals, whereas tolerant animals had fewer. Naor and Sulitzeanu completed the experiment in 1967. Their research led directly to a fundamental question: How could one be sure that the antigen-binding cells were actually the predecessors of the antibody-producing cells?

HOT-ANTIGEN SUICIDE

One of us (Ada), along with Pauline Byrt of the Walter and Eliza Hall Institute of Medical Research in Melbourne, proposed a way to answer that question. If the antibody-producing cells are in fact descended exclusively from the antigen-binding cells, then damaging the ancestral antigen-binding cells by means of a radioactive antigen should prevent the replication of cells producing antibody specific for that antigen. Other cells should not be affected. In 1969 Byrt and Ada went to work on their

so-called hot-antigen-suicide experiments. Two distinct but similar antigens from *Salmonella* bacteria, each one linked with radioactive iodine, where injected into two separate groups of mice. The lymphocytes of those animals were then transferred to two other groups of mice whose own immune systems had been destroyed by X rays. Then both groups of mice were injected with both antigens, this time lacking their radioactive tags. The surrogate immune systems in the irradiated mice secreted few or no antibodies in response to the antigen to which their lymphocytes had been exposed, but they gave the usual robust response to the other antigen. When the antigen-binding cells were crippled, in other words, the immune response to the antigen was crippled as well.

Experiments with hot-antigen suicide gave the clonal-selection theory a significant boost; meanwhile Hans L. R. Wigzell and Birger Andersson of the Karolinska Institute in Stockholm had arrived at similar conclusions using an alternative approach. None of the experiments conducted so far, however, could prove unequivocally that the cell surface bears one and only one kind of receptor. It was clear that the products of an individual cell were less heterogeneous than the serum antibodies, but it was still possible that 10 or 100 specificities, rather than several thousand, were represented on a single cell surface.

In 1973 an ingenious experiment designed by Martin C. Raff, Marc Feldman and Stefanello de Petris of University College London attempted to eliminate this uncertainty. Earlier Raff had discovered a chemical that could cross-link surface receptors on cells. The agent irritates a cell so that all the linked receptors get swept into a tight, caplike section of the cell membrane. A cross-linking substance acting with the specificity of an antigen would cap only those receptors to which it bound. The investigators had such a cross-linking antigen. Would it cap all the receptors on a given cell, or would it leave some behind? Raff and his colleagues applied their cross-linking antigen to white blood cells and found that, on the cells that reacted, more than 95 percent of the receptors had been capped.

PROOF IN THE GELATIN

Now only formal proof was necessary to seal the success of the clonal-selection theory. Scientific rigor called for an experiment that followed a homogeneous population of antigen-binding cells from stimulation by an antigen to replication and antibody production. Until early in the 1970's, however, attempts to prepare a population of healthy cells that were all reactive with just one antigen were frustrating and fruitless. Promising techniques were finally reported by four or five groups; Nossal's laboratory was one of them.

That group came up with a simple method by exploiting the melting properties of gelatin. The workers coupled molecules of a given antigen to gelatin in liquid form and allowed the antigen-gelatin blend to set in shallow dishes. Then 100 million ordinary spleen cells from an unimmunized animal were added to each dish. Cells specific for the embedded antigen would adhere to it; any cells that did not adhere could be washed off. In this way cells reactive with a single antigen were isolated on the gelatin.

The investigators then released the antigen-

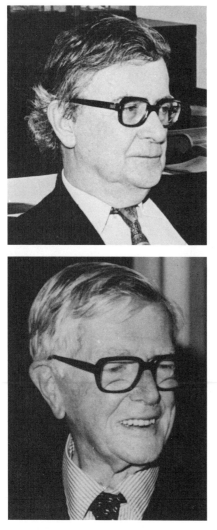
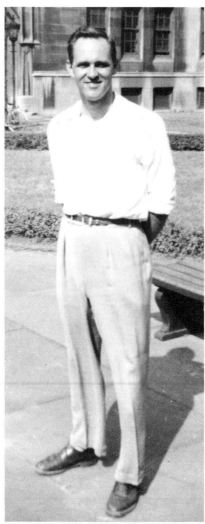

Figure 1.5 THREE ADVOCATES revitalized the selection theory in the 1950's. Niels Kaj Jerne (*top left*) advanced the notion of an antigen as a selective agent; David W. Talmage (*right*) suggested that antigen binding induces antibody-producing cells to replicate. F. Macfarlane Burnet (*bottom left*) maintained that each cell produces just one kind of antibody.

specific cells by melting the gelatin. The antigen was freed from the cells with an enzyme that digests gelatin and pulls the antigen along with it. Once in free solution, each cell was placed in its own culture through techniques developed largely by our colleague Beverley L. Pike of the Walter and Eliza Hall Institute. Each cell was stimulated with the original antigen and a second, irrelevant antigen. As they had expected, Nossal's collaborators found that single cells gave rise to antibody-producing clones in response to the first antigen and not the incidental one. The tissue-culture fluid surrounding the clones was rich with antibodies to the original antigen. The fluid contained no irrelevant antibodies.

THE SCOPE OF SELECTION

Although these cloning experiments were difficult to carry out when they were first reported in 1976, they have since become much more manageable, and the original results have been duplicated many times. Today the concept of clonal selection is accepted as fact, and the direct descent of antibody-producing cells from antigen-binding cells has been firmly established. The antigen-binding cells are the B lymphocytes; their descendants, the antibody-producing clone cells, are known as plasma cells.

We have related this saga as if there had been a simple, direct progression from the conceptualization of the theory to its validation; in truth, the path was much more complex. Many experiments we have not mentioned had tangential but significant impact. The techniques for transferring surrogate immune systems to X-irradiated mice, the unraveling of the structure of the antibody molecule itself and the discovery of the genetic basis for antibody diversity have all contributed to the clonal-selection theory's success.

The last contribution answers a particularly thorny question that dogged the clonal-selection theory: How could lymphocytes anticipate the vast variety of antigens and bear receptors capable of intercepting any one of them? Burnet himself recognized that his theory required some kind of randomization process for which there was no precedent. It is now known that the antigen-binding site of an antibody is the product of no fewer than five different genes, each with several variable regions. The genes recombine as the lymphocyte differentiates, assuming a unique pattern in each cell. That pattern dictates the specificity of the antibodies the cell will produce.

We also chose not to discuss the second great family of lymphocytes, the T cells. These cells defend the body, not by secreting antibodies but by killing infected cells and aiding the process of inflammation. Advances in research on the T lymphocytes have been crucial to completing the picture of the immune system's manifold functions.

Indeed, the process of antibody formation is just one of the many mysteries that have been solved. The immune system is now well understood at the cellular, biochemical and genetic levels. There is still much to learn, but the progress to date augurs well for the future. When the clonal-selection theory of antibody formation was first proposed, it seemed improbable, almost unbelievable. The revolutionary concepts hinted at by Ehrlich and formally developed by Jerne, Talmage and Burnet not only stimulated a vast amount of experimental work but also provided insight into wider aspects of cellular organization and function. The resolution of the problem of antibody origin has influenced vaccine development and organ transplantation as well as protein chemistry and molecular biology. In this respect, the contributions of the scientific trio (see Figure 1.5) who championed the clonal-selection theory must be measured not just within the framework of immunology but within that of biology as a whole.

THE CELLULAR
AND MOLECULAR BASIS
OF IMMUNOLOGICAL SPECIFICITY

. . .

Introduction

The chapters in Section II outline the cellular and molecular basis of immunologic specificity. Antibodies, the blood proteins that are capable of recognizing foreign antigens in extracellular fluids and on cell surfaces, were the first of the recognition structures of the immune system to be discovered. Antibodies, which are proteins designated immunoglobulins, also act as the receptors on the lymphocytes that are the precursors of antibody-producing cells. These cells, the B lymphocytes, express a specialized form of immunoglobulin that contains a membrane-spanning domain, enabling it to function as a cell-surface receptor. When the B cell is stimulated in such a way that it becomes an antibody-secreting cell, the antibody that it secretes has an identical combining specificity to the antibody that acted as its receptor. However, the secreted form of the antibody differs from the receptor in that it lacks the membrane-spanning domain and is, instead, a soluble protein. This change in immunoglobulin structure is achieved through the alternative splicing of RNA to produce mature mRNAs that code for either membrane antibody (receptor) or secreted antibody.

The other major set of lymphocytes, the T lymphocytes, do not produce antibodies, but mediate many important effector functions, such as the killing of virus-infected cells and tumor cells and the production of a set of potent regulatory and effector proteins termed lymphokines or interleukins. The T cells are also the major regulatory cells of the immune system.

T cells possess antigen-specific cell-surface receptors that are similar in many respects to antibodies but display a remarkable and fascinating difference that represents a striking adaptation to their function. Antibodies and T-cell receptors are both members of a large family of molecules with a common set of structural elements referred to as the immunoglobulin supergene family. This family is so designated because immunoglobulins were the first members to be extensively characterized. The basic structural unit of both antibodies and T-cell receptors consists of two distinct polypeptide chains (a heterodimer). For antibodies, one of the two chains is designated the heavy (H) chain and the other the light (L) chain. For the T-cell receptor, the chains are designated alpha and beta (or, for a rare form of the receptor, gamma and delta). Each heterodimer forms an antigen-combining site that is contributed to by amino acids in the N-terminal portion of both chains. These N-terminal regions of the polypeptide chains are designated variable regions because their structures differ when one compares antibodies or T-cell receptors of distinct specificity.

Both the physical nature of the contacts between antibody and antigen and the genetic means through which the enormous variety of different antibodies are created have been solved, representing two of the most impressive accomplishments of modern biological science. Chapter 2, "The Genetics of Antibody Diversity," by Philip Leder, discusses how the generation of antibody diversity is based on a unique genetic mechanism. The coding region for a single immunoglobulin heavy chain variable region (V) is formed by the combinatorial use of genetic elements from three different gene sets—$(V_H$, diversity D and joining $J_H)$—on the same chromosome. This combinatorial process involves gene translocation events in which a single D genetic element is initially brought into apposition with a single J_H element, with the intervening DNA being deleted. Subsequently, a single V_{II} element is apposed to the newly formed D/J_{II} complex, creating the $V_H/D/J_H$ structure. Since there are a large number of different V_H genetic elements (~ 200 in humans), ~ 12 D elements and 4 J_H elements and a substantial degree of randomness in the joining process, the potential number of distinct $V_H/D/J_H$ genes that can be assembled in the cells of a single individual is close to the product of the number of each of these genes (i.e., $\sim 9,600$). Additional diversity is introduced because of an imprecision in the joining process leading to the appearance of codons for different amino acids at the junctions between the regions. Furthermore, new nucleotides may be introduced at the junctions through the action of a specific enzyme, terminal deoxynucleotidyl transferase. These mechanisms thus lead to a further increase in the number of distinct heavy-chain genes that can be created. Light-chain variable region genes are constructed in a similar way although they are made from only V_L and J_L elements; no D elements exist for light chains. Since heavy- and light-chain pairing is, to a large degree, random, the number of distinct heavy-light pairs that can be created is very large indeed, almost certainly well over 10^8.

This process for the creation of the repertoire of antibody genes — the genetic random structure generator, provided by the process of combinatorial association of genetic elements, diversity generation at the junctional regions and combinatorial pairing of heavy and light chains — is not the final word for the creation of diversity for the antibody system. Once an immune response is underway, the cells that are the precursors of antibody-producing cells (B lymphocytes) can activate a process through which a high rate of mutation is induced in the genes specifying heavy- and light-chain variable regions. This process of somatic hypermutation allows the appearance of new antibodies that will occasionally have a higher binding affinity for antigen than the nonmutated antibody. Since B-cell receptors are antibody molecules specialized for expression in membranes, the rare cells that bear such high affinity receptors will have a selective advantage in binding antigen and thus should be selectively stimulated to proliferate. As a result, they should come to dominate the population of antibody-producing cells. The process of affinity maturation of the antibody response leads to the production of antibodies of greater efficiency for the elimination of microorganisms and is a major factor in the resistance to reinfection of individuals who have recovered from infection with a given virus or bacteria or who have been successfully vaccinated against such organisms. One may view the clonal selection of the immune response as having much in common with Darwinian natural selection. Thus, there is a broad array of distinct individuals (cells) encompassing a large pool of distinct genes; a powerful selective system introduced by microorganisms with antigens capable of stimulating the growth of only those cells with complementary receptors, and a subsequent mutational diversification process capable of introducing new genetic diversity among the selected individuals. However, rather than involving selection of individual organisms as a result of the action of products of genes in the germ line, occurring over many generations, clonal selection involves selection among somatic cells during the life of a single animal. This process of somatic evolution of the immune system seems very well-suited to allow higher organisms to develop responses capable of meeting the antigenic challenge posed by the rapid potential for conventional evolution possessed by microorganisms.

Antibodies, although key elements in responses against many microorganisms, are largely limited in their protective function to organisms that are found in extracellular fluid or on the surfaces of cells. The other major element of the immune system, the T cells, are specialized to deal with antigens that are cell-associated, including products of viruses and bacteria that are obligatory intracellular pathogens. Immunity mediated by T lymphocytes is often referred to as cellular immunity.

The specialized function of T lymphocytes is to a large degree implicit in the unusual specificity of their receptors. T-cell receptors are heterodimers of alpha and beta (or gamma and delta) chains that have many features in common with antibodies, including the genetic mechanisms for the generation of diversity, with the exception of somatic hypermutation. T cells do not appear to use somatic hypermutation at least in part to avoid difficulties in the maintenance of immunological tolerance.

However, as discussed in Chapter 3, "The T Cell and Its Receptor," by Philippa Marrack and John Kappler, and in Chapter 4, "How T Cells See Antigen," by Howard M. Grey, Alessandro Sette, and Søren Buus, the structure of antigens recognized by T cells differs in a key way from those recognized by antibodies. T-cell receptors are not specific for soluble molecules in free solution or for structures displayed on the surface of microorganisms. Rather, they recognize a molecular complex consisting of a peptide, derived from a foreign molecule, and a specialized cell surface protein of the host, either a class I or class II major histocompatibility complex (MHC) molecule. The peptide component of this complex is derived, by proteolysis, from proteins either taken into the cell by endocytosis or produced within the cell. This peptide is bound into a specialized groove in class I or class II MHC molecules and is brought to the cell surface with the MHC molecule. The interaction between the peptide and the MHC groove is a specific one. Only certain peptides bind to given forms of MHC class I or class II molecules, determining which portions of a protein are immunogenic or, indeed, whether some proteins are immunogenic or not. MHC molecules display a high degree of variation from individual to individual. Indeed, their structural polymorphism is one reason why immune responses to them are central to the rejection of organ and tissue grafts between non-identical individuals. For this reason, these molecules are often referred to as transplantation antigens. Many of the amino acids that vary between individuals are found in the groove of the MHC molecules and are believed to be contact residues in the binding of peptides to class I and class II MHC molecules. For this reason, individuals of distinct MHC type often recognize different peptides and consequently different portions of a given protein. In some circumstances, this difference in peptide-binding capacity of different polymorphic forms of MHC class I or class II molecules will lead to genetically determined differences in capacity to mount immune responses to specific antigens. When such differences were first appreciated and were shown to be controlled by genes in the MHC region, the genes were referred to as immune-response genes.

MHC molecules are largely specialized in that class I MHC molecules principally bind peptides from proteins produced within a cell, such as peptides derived from viral proteins or possibly proteins in tumor cells that possess mutations, such as oncogene products. By contrast, class II MHC molecules principally bind peptides derived from extracellular proteins that have entered the cell through endocytosis. Indeed, T cells can be divided into two subtypes, marked by the expression of the cell surface molecules CD4 and CD8. These cell surface markers determine whether a T cell is specialized to recognize peptides associated with class I or class II MHC molecules, to a large degree because the CD4 protein binds to class II molecules and the CD8 protein binds to class I MHC molecules.

The specificity of T cells for complexes of antigen-derived peptides and obligatory cell surface molecules (class I and class II MHC molecules) ensures that T cells recognize antigens on the surface of other cells. Such spatial constraint in recognition is critically associated with T-cell function since T cells do not act directly on pathogenic agents but rather act on other cell types, most particularly cells that have either bound foreign antigens or cells that are infected with foreign organisms. Such localized recognition ensures that the T cell will become activated at the site of cells bearing antigen or infected with particular infectious agents. T cells will thus mediate their function, whether to help B cells make

specific antibodies, to enable macrophages to destroy microorganisms they have ingested, or to kill virus infected cells, precisely in the context of the affected cells.

The capacity to recognize peptides derived from proteins produced by cells, such as viral proteins or endogenous proteins that have mutated, can extend T-cell surveillance to proteins that are not, in their intact form, expressed on the cell surface. Thus, the T-cell recognition strategy allows the T cells to monitor antigens that are normally regarded as obligatory intracellular molecules. As an analogy, one may say that the peptide recognition mechanism provides the T-cell system with the equivalent of a fiber optic scope to peer inside of living cells.

One may also consider both repertoire acquisition and induction of immunologic tolerance in T cells in terms of their unique pattern of receptor specificity. There is now strong evidence that the peripheral T-cell population of mice is derived by a developmental process within the thymus, in which T cells are positively selected by virtue of having receptors that recognize antigen-derived peptides bound to MHC molecules of the same polymorphic form possessed by the responding individual. At the same time T cells that can bind a self-antigen, associated with self-MHC molecules, are often eliminated, particularly when the complex of self-antigen and self-MHC molecules are found within the thymus. Recent work has directly demonstrated both clonal deletion of T cells capable of strong reactivity with self-antigens and self-MHC molecules, as well as the positive selection of T cells capable of responding to self-MHC molecules. It is not clear what determines whether a given encounter within the thymus will lead to tolerance induction or to thymic selection. This is a central area of contemporary research and one that should have great importance for the future.

When the expanded diversification of the B cell receptor system, accomplished by somatic hypermutation, is coupled with an antigen-driven selection process, a marked increase occurs in the effectiveness of antibody in the course of the immune response. T cells do not appear to use somatic hypermutation to provide the opportunity for progressive selection of receptors that are better fitted to their cognate antigens. Analysis of sequences of T-cell receptor genes at various times after the initiation of the response does not reveal the occurrence of mutation. It has been suggested that T cells do not employ somatic mutation for diversification after interaction with antigen because such diversification might, by chance, lead to the appearance of T cells that can recognize and respond to self-antigens, thus frustrating the process through which tolerance had been originally established. Such an explanation is only tenable, however, if the danger to the organism from autoreactive antibodies would be less severe than the danger from autoreactive T cells or if autoreactive B cells would not be stimulated to produce antibody without autoreactive T

cells. Indeed, there is reason to believe that both of these possibilities are correct, indicting that somatic hypermutation could be more easily allowed among B-cell receptors (antibodies) than among T-cell receptors.

The three chapters of Section II should provide the reader with a picture of the exciting progress being made in the field of the molecular and cellular basis of immunologic recognition.

The Genetics of Antibody Diversity

Segments of DNA and RNA are shuffled and joined in various ways as cells of the immune system develop. The combinatorial process can generate information specifying billions of different antibodies.

· · ·

Philip Leder
May, 1982

The immune system of a vertebrate animal has a virtually unlimited capacity to generate different antibodies, which recognize and bind to many millions of potential antigens, or "nonself" molecules. This implies that many millions of species of antibody molecules are synthesized by the cells of the immune system. An antibody is an assembly of protein chains, and the structure of a protein chain is specified by a unit of genetic information: a gene. Hence it would seem there must be many millions of antibody genes. Yet the genome, or total genetic complement, of a mammal amounts to perhaps a million genes, and only a small fraction of them can specify antibodies. The paradox of a limited number of genes and an apparently limitless capacity to generate different antibodies has been a major puzzle for immunologists and geneticists for more than two decades. The solution of the puzzle is now emerging. It represents both a dramatic confluence of the two disciplines and an early triumph of some remarkable new techniques of molecular genetics.

In essence the answer is that the genes ultimately specifying the structure of each antibody are not present as such in germ cells (the male sperm and the female egg) or in the cells of the early embryo.

Rather than harboring a set of complete and active antibody genes, these cells contain bits and pieces of the genes: a kit of components. The components are shuffled in the cells of the immune system called *B* lymphocytes as those cells develop and mature. The shuffling can lead to a different result in each of millions of lines of cells. Individual mutations amplify the diversity. The result is that in the mature descendants of each line a unique gene is assembled, whose information is expressed in the form of a unique antibody.

PROTEINS AND GENES

Antibodies, like other proteins, are made up of the subunits called amino acids. There are 20 kinds of amino acids, which can be linked together in any combination to form a protein chain. The amino acid composition of a chain and the sequence in which the amino acids are arrayed along the chain determine how the chain folds in three dimensions and perhaps combines with other chains. Substituting one amino acid for another or altering the sequence changes the protein's properties.

The amino acid composition and sequence of a protein chain are prescribed by a gene, which is a segment of another kind of chain: a molecule of the nucleic acid DNA, the hereditary material of the cell. The subunits of DNA are four nucleotides, each of which is characterized by one of four chemical bases: adenine (A), guanine (G), thymine (T) and cytosine (C). The nucleotides are assembled to form a strand of DNA, and the sequence of their bases along the strand defines the information carried by the gene. The information is deciphered by means of the genetic code, whose code words (called codons) are triplets of bases: CTG, say, or AGC. In general each codon specifies an amino acid, and a long series of codons supplies instructions for assembling an entire protein chain consisting of hundreds of amino acids. The information in DNA is not translated directly into a protein, however. First it is transcribed into a single strand of the similar nucleic acid RNA. The new informational molecule, which is called messenger RNA, is translated into protein.

In higher organisms the genetic information for most proteins is not arranged in a continuous sequence of DNA codons. Instead most genes are split: patches of coding sequences are separated by noncoding intervening sequences. A split gene is first transcribed, noncoding segments and all, into RNA. Then the primary transcript is spliced: the intervening sequences are eliminated and the coding sequences are joined to form a coherent messenger RNA.

Immunoglobulins, the antibody molecules, have structural features that reflect their function. An antibody molecule is made up of two kinds of related protein chains, designated light and heavy (see Figure 2.1). When the amino acid sequences of light chains from various antibodies were compared almost two decades ago by Norbert Hilschmann, who was then working at the Rockefeller Institute for Medical Research, he found that the chains have a peculiar property. The sequences of chains from

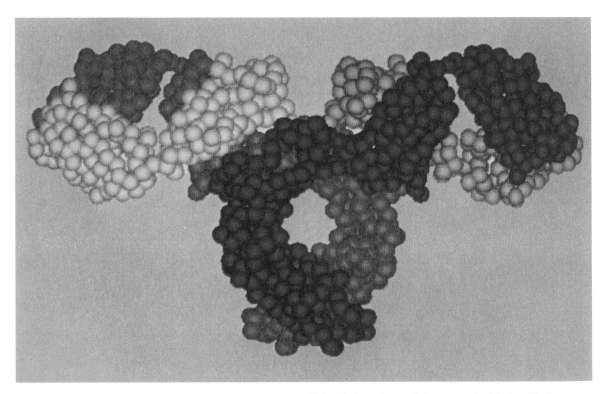

Figure 2.1 ANTIBODY MOLECULE is an assembly of four protein chains, which are folded and interconnected to form a split *T*. There are two identical heavy chains (*red and dark blue*) and two identical light chains (*yellow and light blue*). In this model, generated with the aid of a computer by Richard J. Feldmann, the spheres represent amino acids, the subunits of the protein chains.

different antibodies are different from one another, but the differences are confined to the first half of each chain. The remainder of the chain has essentially the same sequence in all antibodies of a given type.

A BIFUNCTIONAL MOLECULE

The presence of both variation and constancy in a single protein molecule turned out to have great functional significance. Indeed, an antibody is a bifunctional molecule (see Figure 2.2). Each chain has a variable region (about half of a light chain and about one-fourth of a heavy chain) and a constant region. It is the variable regions of the chains that fold up in space to form an antibody-antigen combining site: the site that binds to the particular anti-gen against which the antibody is directed. Changing the amino acid sequence in the variable region changes the combining site's chemical structure and thereby changes the affinity of the antibody for an antigen, much as altering a notch on the serrated part of a key makes it fit a different lock.

The constant region of an antibody's light and heavy chains is analogous to the handle of a key, which is identical from one key to another of a given make and type and serves a function common to all keys. The constant region of an antibody molecule of a particular type serves the same function in every molecule of that type. For example, there are two types of light chain in most vertebrate animals, kappa and lambda; every antibody molecule must have light chains of one type or the other. In any species the constant region of each kappa or

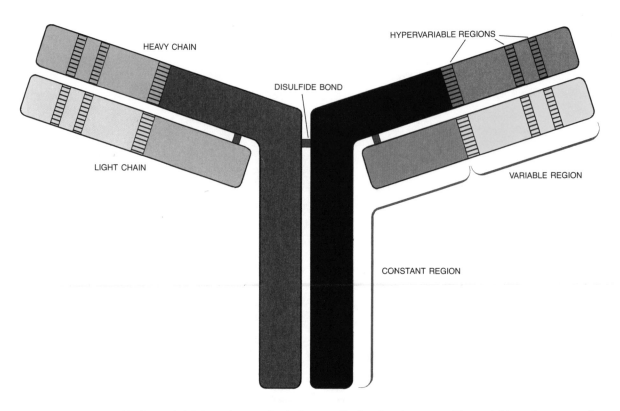

Figure 2.2 BIFUNCTIONAL NATURE of an antibody is reflected in its structure, as is seen in this schematic diagram of the molecule modeled in Figure 2.1. Each protein chain has a variable region and a constant region. In the variable regions the sequence of amino acids is different in each antibody; the constant regions are the same in every antibody of a given type. The variable regions recognize and bind to a specific antigen; the constant regions thereupon carry out some immunologic task. The chains are folded so that their hypervariable regions, where the amino acid sequence is particularly variable, come together to form a highly specific antigen-combining site.

lambda light chain is identical with the constant region of other chains of the same type.

In addition each antibody molecule has one of five heavy-chain types: mu, delta, gamma, epsilon or alpha. The heavy-chain type defines the class of the immunoglobulin as IgM, IgD, IgG, IgE or IgA. In secreted antibodies of the IgM class, for example, all the heavy chains have the same mu constant-region sequence and all the light chains have the same kappa or lambda constant-region sequence. Their variable regions, on the other hand, differ from one antibody to the next, reflecting their different antigenic specificities.

The constant region of the heavy chains determines the effector function of an antibody, or how it carries out its immunologic task in the body. Consider an antibody whose variable region is specific for an antigen found on ragweed pollen. If the heavy chain is of the delta type, the IgD antibody it forms remains associated with the surface of the cell that makes it. If the gamma heavy chain is present, the resulting IgG antibody is likely to circulate in the blood. If the epsilon chain is present, the antibody (IgE) may bind to the surface of a specialized cell that releases histamine, giving rise to the symptoms of hay fever or asthma when the antibody interacts with the ragweed antigen. All the antibodies are specific for the same antigen, namely the ragweed one. Furthermore, the same effector functions are found in antibodies directed against other antigens; the effector function is independent of the variable region.

THE DREYER-BENNETT HYPOTHESIS

It was the structural features of antibodies that offered the first clues to the genetic source of their diversity. William J. Dreyer and J. Claude Bennett, who were working at the California Institute of Technology in the mid-1960's, recognized that a million different antibodies could be generated by combining 1,000 different light chains with 1,000 different heavy chains. Nevertheless, Dreyer and Bennett wondered how the genetic information for this diversity of proteins could be organized. Above all, what organization could account for the strange variable-and-constant structure of each chain?

Consider just the problem of one type of light chain. There might conceivably be 1,000 genes, each gene specifying one of 1,000 light chains. In that case, however, some mechanism must have operated in the course of evolution to preserve un-

changed the sequence of the constant-region half of each of the 1,000 genes while the other half of each gene (the half encoding the variable region) was allowed to mutate widely. Such a mechanism seemed unlikely because there is no obvious biological reason for any given constant-region amino acid sequence to have been conserved. Comparisons of immunoglobulins in different individuals and species indicate there is little evolutionary pressure to maintain absolute identity among constant-region sequences; a change of a few amino acids in the constant region seems to have no ill effect.

Dreyer and Bennett made a radical proposal. Instead of assuming that the genetic information for an antibody light chain is specified by a continuous array of codons, they proposed that the light chain is encoded in two discontinuous stretches of DNA, one for the variable region and the other for the constant region. Moreover, they proposed that there are several hundred or several thousand separately encoded variable-region genes in the DNA of germ cells but only one constant-region gene.

By postulating a single constant-region gene, the Dreyer-Bennett proposal showed how essentially the same sequence might be conserved to appear in every constant region of a given type in a given species. If there is only one constant-region gene, any mutation in it must immediately alter the amino acid sequence of every light chain. Also implicit in the proposal was the notion that the information in the separate genetic elements must somehow come together to form a contiguous and coherent genetic message and then a single protein chain. The proposal of Dreyer and Bennett initially attracted considerable criticism; it called for split genes and for mechanisms to join them, both of which were then quite without precedent. Yet the idea proved to be essentially correct.

EARLY EXPERIMENTS

In 1971 I set to work with my colleague David C. Swan at the National Institute of Child Health and Human Development to test the Dreyer-Bennett hypothesis. Our strategy was to detect and isolate the initial product of an antibody gene: its messenger RNA. A strand of DNA artificially copied from that messenger (by means of the enzyme reverse transcriptase) would serve as a probe with which to detect the antibody genes in embryonic cells and estimate how many such genes are present. This would enable us to test the central prediction of the

Dreyer-Bennett hypothesis: that there is only one constant-region gene, or at the most a few, as opposed to the many genes required by the more straightforward genetic models.

We used the technique of hybridization kinetics. Two stretches of nucleic acid with complementary nucleotide sequences are able to hybridize, or bind to each other. If one of the sequences has been labeled with atoms of a radioactive isotope, the hybrid molecules can be identified by their radioactivity. The speed with which a radioactive DNA probe finds and hybridizes with any complementary DNA molecules (the hybridization kinetics) is an indirect but effective measure of the number of such complementary molecules in the preparation. We measured the rate at which our probe (DNA copied from the RNA specifying the constant region of the mouse light chain) hybridized with DNA representing the entire genome of the mouse embryo. With the help of Tasuku Honjo, who had joined us from Kyoto University, we got results indicating clearly that there are very few copies of the light-chain constant-region gene, perhaps no more than two in each cell. Similar results were soon obtained in a number of other laboratories. Clearly the Dreyer-Bennett hypothesis had to be taken seriously.

If there are only a few copies of the constant-region gene and many separately encoded variable-region genes, some mechanism must operate to bring the information together in a coherent sequence. The most economical way to bring this about would be at the level of the gene, that is, to join two sequences of DNA that are separate in an embryonic cell to form a single active sequence in the nucleus of a mature, antibody-producing lymphocyte. Such a rearrangement of the DNA in the course of the differentiation and development of somatic, or body, cells is referred to as somatic recombination. The discovery of the enzymes called restriction endonucleases, which cleave DNA at specific sites, paved the way for an important experiment testing the notion of somatic recombination.

Susumu Tonegawa and Nobumichi Hozumi of the Basel Institute for Immunology compared DNA from the mouse embryo with DNA from a plasmacytoma: a tumor composed of plasma cells, or mature B lymphocytes, that produce antibody molecules of a single type and specificity (see Figure 2.3). Cells from these tumors, most of which have been prepared by Michael Potter of the National Cancer Institute, serve to provide the investigator with a large quantity of a particular antibody and of the DNA and RNA that encode it; the cells have been invaluable in many lines of immunologic research.

Tonegawa and Hozumi reasoned that if the DNA surrounding the antibody genes had undergone somatic recombination in the tumor's antibody-producing cells, it should be arranged differently from the DNA of embryonic cells. The difference would be reflected in the spacing of the sites that are cut by a given restriction endonuclease. For example, if the constant-region gene in embryonic DNA is surrounded by two restriction sites (sites cleaved by a particular endonuclease) 5,000 nucleotides apart, after the cleavage the gene is found embedded in a fragment of DNA 5,000 nucleotides long. If somatic recombination eliminates one of the sites and brings in a new one, the plasmacytoma DNA may yield a constant-region fragment either longer or shorter than 5,000 nucleotides. Tonegawa and Hozumi were able to show that the arrangement of light-chain genes is different in embryonic cells and antibody-producing cells. The activation of the genes in the course of development is accompanied by their somatic recombination: the genes are shuffled.

CLONING

The mid-1970's was a period of extraordinary developments in molecular genetics, accompanied by some controversy and misunderstanding. A major advance, in 1973, was the first successful application of new recombinant-DNA techniques to insert foreign DNA into a bacterium or a bacterial virus and thereby clone a single gene in quantity. It was immediately clear to those of us working with more cumbersome genetic techniques that gene cloning would enable us to isolate antibody genes and determine their structure in a direct way. There was uncertainty, however, about possible hazards of the procedures; the safety of the methods has since been established, but at that time the National Institutes of Health promulgated cautious guidelines for recombinant-DNA experiments. Among the requirements were some that affected vector organisms: the bacteria or bacterial viruses in which foreign DNA is cloned. The vector had to be genetically crippled to reduce its chance of survival outside the laboratory by a factor of 100 million.

My colleagues David C. Tiemeier, Lynn Enquist, Nathan Sternberg, Robert A. Weisberg and I decided to adapt the bacteriophage, or bacterial virus,

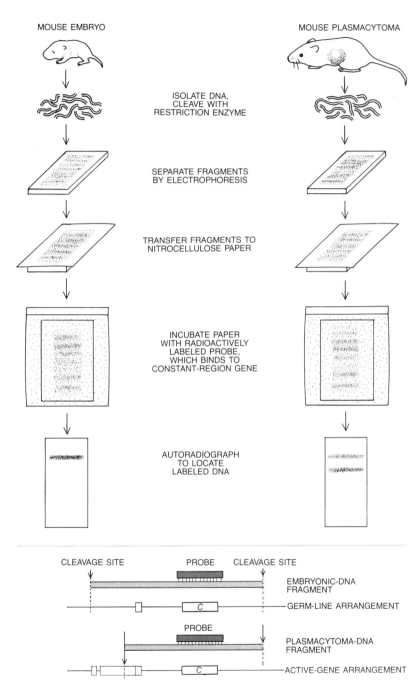

MOUSE EMBRYO

MOUSE PLASMACYTOMA

ISOLATE DNA,
CLEAVE WITH
RESTRICTION ENZYME

SEPARATE FRAGMENTS
BY ELECTROPHORESIS

TRANSFER FRAGMENTS TO
NITROCELLULOSE PAPER

INCUBATE PAPER
WITH RADIOACTIVELY
LABELED PROBE,
WHICH BINDS TO
CONSTANT-REGION GENE

AUTORADIOGRAPH
TO LOCATE
LABELED DNA

CLEAVAGE SITE   PROBE   CLEAVAGE SITE

EMBRYONIC-DNA
FRAGMENT

C   GERM-LINE ARRANGEMENT

PROBE

PLASMACYTOMA-DNA
FRAGMENT

C   ACTIVE-GENE ARRANGEMENT

Figure 2.3 GENE SHUFFLING demonstrated by comparing DNA fragments on which a constant-region gene (C) is found in a mouse embryo and a plasmacytoma. A restriction enzyme cleaves the DNA at specific sites, and the fragments are separated and identified with a probe (color) that binds to any DNA having a largely complementary nucleotide sequence. The embryonic DNA yields one radioactive band, which corresponds to a single fragment carrying the C gene in its germ-line configuration. The plasmacytoma DNA yields two bands. One band represents the germ-line configuration, which is maintained by one of two versions of the gene (alleles) in the antibody-producing cell, and the other band represents the other allele, which carries the C sequence in the rearranged configuration of an active antibody gene.

called phage lambda for this purpose. A version of the phage engineered by Ronald W. Davis of the Stanford University School of Medicine could be genetically rigged so that it would grow only if it had picked up a piece of foreign DNA. We introduced a series of crippling mutations into the phage vector, carried out appropriate survival tests and ultimately received the necessary approval. Soon Shirley M. Tilghman, Tiemeier and I were able to report the first successful cloning in a bacteriophage of a mammalian gene: a mouse gene for globin (the protein of the hemoglobin molecule).

In response to a request from Tonegawa's laboratory we sent a supply of our disabled phage to Switzerland, where the cloning strategy was exploited by Tonegawa and his colleagues to isolate the mouse genes for the lambda light chain in both embryonic and antibody-producing cells. They discovered that the constant-region gene and the variable-region genes are indeed encoded far apart in the DNA of cells that do not synthesize antibodies. In an appropriate antibody-producing plasmacytoma the two genes are much closer together. The rearrangement does not, however, bring the variable-region and the constant-region genes together to form a continuous sequence. Instead, the variable-region gene (V) is still about 1,500 nucleotides away from the constant-region gene (C); between them, and abutting the V gene, is a segment called the J (for joining) sequence, as I shall explain below.

Our own cloning efforts were directed toward the kappa light-chain genes of the mouse. We undertook to examine this system because more than 95 percent of mouse antibodies incorporate the kappa chain, making it the major source of mouse light-chain diversity. My colleagues Jonathan G. Seidman and Edward E. Max cloned both the embryonic and the active forms of the kappa variable-region and constant-region genes. Then, by means of the rapid DNA-sequencing technique developed by Alan Maxam and Walter Gilbert of Harvard University, they determined the nucleotide sequences of the genes.

THE KAPPA CHAIN

A large number of V genes were identified in the embryonic DNA. They seem to fall into families, each family being made up of genes whose nucleotide sequences are closely related. Our own studies and those of Robert P. Perry of the Institute for Cancer Research in Fox Chase, Pa., indicate that as many as several hundred variable-region genes may

be present in mouse-embryo DNA. Each of the V genes, whether kappa or lambda, retains certain structural features that appear to be of considerable significance. For example, each gene is divided into two discrete coding segments separated by a short intervening sequence. The first coding sequence specifies a hydrophobic (water-repellent) "leader," 17 to 20 amino acids long, that is thought to be important for the transport of the antibody molecule through the cell membrane. The leader is a part of the original protein product of the active light-chain gene but is cleaved away as the nascent antibody passes through the membrane (see Figure 2.4).

The other coding region of the V gene specifies most of the variable region, but not all of it. The nonleader part of the V gene encodes only 95 of the 108 amino acids of the kappa chain's variable region. As Tonegawa's earlier findings had suggested was the case in the lambda system, we found that in the kappa DNA the remaining portion of the variable region is encoded by a sequence well "downstream" from the V gene, near the single constant-region gene, exactly at the site to which the V gene is joined to make an active immunoglobulin gene. This short sequence, the J gene, is repeated with slight but significant variations five times at intervals of about 300 nucleotides. (In the mouse lambda system further studies by Tonegawa, David Baltimore of the Massachusetts Institute of Technology and Ursula Storb of the University of Washington have shown that the arrangement is somewhat different. Instead of one constant-region gene there are four C genes, each with its own J gene. In the human lambda system, Philip A. Hieter, Gregory F. Hollis and I have found, there are six C genes.)

Now the potential of the kappa system to develop diversity begins to come clear. The joining of one of several hundred V genes—say 150 to be conservative—to one of five J genes can generate 150 × 5, or 750, different active genes for a light-chain variable region. Evidence from a number of laboratories indicates that this is exactly the way the sequences are shuffled. One of the V genes is joined to one of the J genes; the extra V's and J's (and the long noncoding spacer) between them are deleted. The finished active gene is encoded in three separate coding sequences: a leader gene, a V/J gene and a C gene. The sequences are assembled by RNA splicing to form a coherent light-chain messenger RNA.

The 750-fold diversity I have accounted for is multiplied by another source of variation. Careful comparisons of the amino acid sequences of light

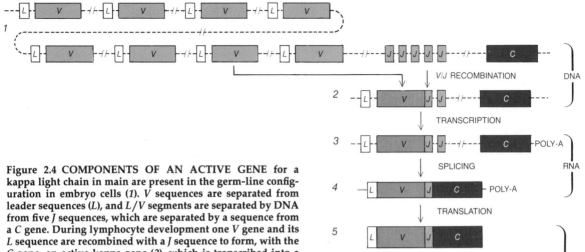

Figure 2.4 COMPONENTS OF AN ACTIVE GENE for a kappa light chain in main are present in the germ-line configuration in embryo cells (*1*). *V* sequences are separated from leader sequences (*L*), and *L/V* segments are separated by DNA from five *J* sequences, which are separated by a sequence from a *C* gene. During lymphocyte development one *V* gene and its *L* sequence are recombined with a *J* sequence to form, with the *C* gene, an active kappa gene (*2*), which is transcribed into a primary RNA transcript (*3*). The intervening sequences and any extra *J*'s are spliced out to yield a coherent messenger RNA (*4*), which is translated into the light-chain percursor (*5*). Leader is cleaved away as mature chain (*6*) passes through cell membranes.

chains revealed a particularly high degree of diversity in a region close to the site of *V/J* joining. The amino acids around position 96 form one of the three regions of the light chains that Elvin A. Kabat of the College of Physicians and Surgeons of Columbia University had earlier designated as "hypervariable." The light chains fold up in such a way that the hypervariable regions form the antibody-antigen combining site.

At least some part of the variation in this region can now be explained by the fact that the *V/J* recombination site is not precisely defined. A *V* gene and a *J* gene can apparently be joined at different crossover points (see Figure 2.5). As a result the codon for amino acid 96 (the nominal *V/J* junction) and the codons adjacent to it can change depending on what part of the sequence is supplied by the embryonic *V* region and what part by the *J* region. If one makes the assumption that alternative joining sites can increase the diversity tenfold, the total number of potential *V/J* combinations becomes 150 × 5 × 10, or 7,500.

SIGNAL SEQUENCES

I mentioned above that certain features of the sequences of the light-chain genes have been conserved and seem likely to be of functional significance. In particular a pattern of signal-like

sequences is found on the so-called 3', or downstream, side of the *V* genes and on the 5', or upstream, side of the *J* genes. Each such sequence has a stretch of about nine nucleotides (a nonamer) of which a large proportion are either A's or T's. The nonamer is followed, at an interval of either about 11 or about 22 nucleotides, by a seven-nucleotide sequence, or heptamer: CACTGTG or GTGACAC. The nonamer and the heptamer can be visualized as forming a "stem" structure in which the sequences would be complementary according to the rules of base pairing (A pairs with T, G with C), bringing the *V* and the *J* genes together at the base of the stem (see Figure 2.6). It is then easy to see how the genes might be joined by some kind of DNA-recombination mechanism, with the signal sequences being deleted. The process is probably mediated by a specific (but as yet undiscovered) system of recombinatory enzymes.

The flexibility of the recombinational system, although powerful in its ability to generate diversity, does have its price. *V* and *J* genes are occasionally brought together aberrantly, yielding an inactive gene. This fact may in part explain the phenomenon called allelic exclusion. Each somatic cell has two sets of chromosomes, with one member of each chromosome pair supplied by the mother and the other by the father. The corresponding copies of a given gene on the two chromosomes are called al-

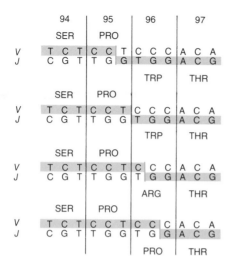

Figure 2.5 RECOMBINATIONAL FLEXIBILITY amplifies antibody diversity. The crossover point (*dark colored lines*) at which the *V* and the *J* sequences recombine can vary over a range of several nucleotides, giving rise to different nucleotide sequences (*colored bands*) in the active kappa-chain gene. The result is that the codon for amino acid 96 of the chain can vary: TGG codes for the amino acid tryptophan, CGG for arginine and CCG for proline. The variation is within the third hypervariable region of the kappa chain, and so it can have a large effect on the antigen-combining site.

leles. In an antibody-producing cell it is usually the case that only the antibody genes on one copy of the chromosome carrying such genes undergo somatic recombination and are finally translated into protein; the alleles on the other chromosome are ordinarily excluded from the rearrangement process and are not expressed. Occasionally, however, an antibody-producing cell has two sets of rearranged antibody genes. My colleagues and I suspect that in such cases the genes on one chromosome were recombined aberrantly, forming an inactive antibody gene, and that the active gene was thereupon generated in a second try, with the "spare" chromosome serving as the backup.

It is also possible that the lambda light-chain genes serve as a fail-safe system for misjoined kappa genes. Studies done by Hieter, Hollis, Stanley J. Korsmeyer, Thomas A. Waldmann and me show that there is a clear order of events in the formation of a light-chain gene. First the kappa genes rearrange. If the kappa genes fail to form an active gene, the lambda system begins to rearrange.

Baltimore and his co-workers at MIT have proposed the intriguing notion that the appearance of a functional antibody in a cell acts as a signal precluding further *V/J* joining; in the absence of the signal the cell keeps trying. In human beings, with six lambda *J/C* sequences on each chromosome No. 22, there are in effect 12 lambda genes per cell. Together with the two kappa genes (one on each chromosome No. 2), that would mean the cell has 14 opportunities to form an active light-chain gene.

THE HEAVY CHAIN

In the heavy chain the formation of the variable region is governed by the same principles that apply in the light chain, but the potential for diversity is even greater: an extra piece of genetic information multiples the combinatorial possibilities. When Leroy E. Hood and his colleagues at Cal Tech cloned an antibody-producing cell's active heavy-chain variable-region DNA and determined its structure, they found that a sequence of at least 13 nucleotides exactly at the *V/J* junction could not be accounted for by either the *V* or the *J* genes in the embryonic DNA. They reasoned that this segment must be supplied by a stretch of embryonic DNA they called the *D* (for diversity) gene. They noted that the *D* segment's location in the active gene corresponds to the major portion of the third hypervariable region of the heavy chain.

Philip W. Early and Hood also noted in the embryonic heavy-chain DNA the nonamer-heptamer sequences that seem to serve in light-chain DNA as signals for *V/J* joining. The arrangement of those signals in light-chain DNA had indicated that the spacing between the nonamer and the heptamer had to be different on the *V* side and the *J* side of the stem structure (about 11 nucleotides on one side and about 22 on the other) for recombination to take place. In the heavy chain, however, the *V* and the *J* signals were both found to have spacers about 22 nucleotides long. Early and Hood therefore predicted that when the *D* genes were identified in

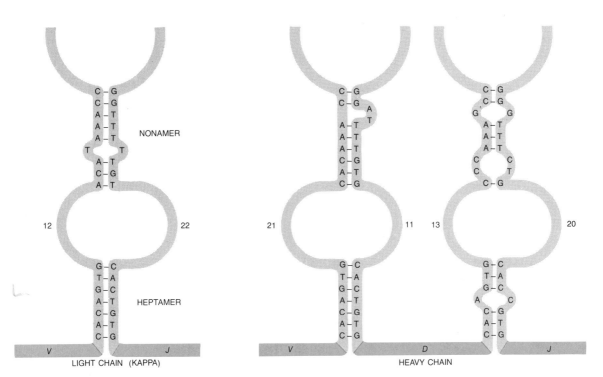

Figure 2.6 RECOMBINATION SIGNALS in germ-line DNA apparently serve to bring *V* and *J* sequences for the light chain together prior to recombination. For the heavy chain a similar mechanism operates, but it includes signals for the *D* (diversity) sequence. The hepatmer and nonamer are separated by a spacer roughly 11 or 22 nucleotides long. Two signal segments whose heptamers and nonamers are largely complementary according to the rules for base pairing (A pairs with T and G pairs with C) might form a stem structure that brings the coding sequences adjoining them together for recombination. Apparently the recombination takes place only when one of the two complementary signals has a short spacer and the other signal has a long spacer.

embryonic DNA, they would be found to be flanked by recombination signals having the 11-nucleotide spacing. In this way the joining of *V* to *D* and of *D* to *J* would conform to the 11/22 rule.

The putative *D* segments presented a problem in cloning. Their coding sequences were too short for them to serve as a hybridization probe for detecting their embryonic counterparts. My colleagues Ulrich Siebenlist and Jeffrey V. Ravetch solved the problem by taking advantage of an aberrant intermediate product of *V/D/J* recombination: a human *D* segment that had somehow been joined incorrectly to a *J* gene. The *D* gene had been processed by the recombinatory enzymes on only one side (the side next to the *J* gene), and so its opposite flank carried with it a large segment of embryonic DNA. The aberrant segment made an excellent probe for cloning embryonic *D* sequences.

When Siebenlist and Ravetch determined the structure of the DNA in these clones, the *D* sequences were found to be surrounded by recombination signals with 11-nucleotide spacers, fulfilling the predictions of the 11/22 rule. Then, with the cloned *D* segment as a probe, Siebenlist and Ravetch searched the human genome for sequences with which it would hybridize. They detected a large *D*-gene family consisting of at least five closely related sequences. There are indications that this is only one of several such families of *D* genes.

The formation of the active gene for the heavy-chain variable region can generate an extraordinarily large number of genetic possibilities (see Figure 2.7). T. H. Rabbitts and his colleagues at the Medical Research Council Laboratory of Molecular Biology in Cambridge have estimated that there are as many as 80 embryonic heavy-chain *V* genes in man. Ravetch has found six active *J* genes within 8,000 nucleotides of the human mu *C* gene. Although one cannot confidently extrapolate the number of human *D* genes from what is known now, I shall assume that the *D* families have about 50 members. Somatic recombination can thus generate approximately $80 \times 6 \times 50$, or 24,000, genetic combinations. Another factor of about 100 (a very rough estimate) is contributed by recombinational flexibility: alternative codons at the two crossover points of *V/D* and *D/J* recombination. The total then comes to about 2.4 million possible different heavy chains.

18 BILLION ANTIBODIES

Taken together with the 7,500 combinatorial possibilities available to the human kappa light chain (150 for the complement of *V* genes, five for the *J* genes and 10 for recombinational flexibility), the 2.4 million heavy chains yield a total of some 18 billion (2.4 million multiplied by 7,500) possible antibodies. They can be generated from perhaps 300 separate genetic segments in the embryonic DNA.

The enormous diversity generated by means of recombination may be supplemented by yet another mechanism: solitary somatic mutation, which introduces sporadic single-nucleotide changes throughout the variable-region DNA in the course of somatic development. Immunoglobulin genes are highly unstable in antibody-producing cells. When Matthew D. Scharff and his colleagues at the Albert Einstein College of Medicine propagated clones of mature lymphocytes and screened successive generations for new antigen-binding specificity, they found the immunoglobulin genes underwent mutation at the remarkable rate of once per 10,000 cells per generation. In other experiments active genes have been isolated whose variable-region DNA differs by one nucleotide or two from the embryonic-DNA sequences that were its source.

These findings support the suggestion, made by Melvin Cohn and Martin Weigert of the Salk Institute for Biological Studies about 15 years ago, that some proportion of antibody diversity is the result of single-nucleotide mutation in the variable-region DNA of developing lymphocytes. Patricia J. Gearhart of the Carnegie Institution of Washington and Hood and Baltimore and their associates have evidence to suggest that the mutations accumulate as the lymphocyte passes through progressive stages in its development. The mechanism that leads to such mutations is not known.

CONSTANT-REGION SHUFFLING

The gene shuffling that can generate billions of variable-region genes is matched by two additional processes that explain how a single variable region can be joined successively to a series of heavy-chain constant regions (see Figure 2.8). A precursor of the antibody-producing cells, the pre-*B* lymphocyte, makes a mu heavy-chain constant region linked to a

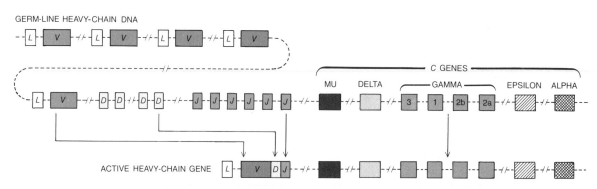

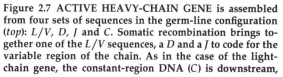

Figure 2.7 ACTIVE HEAVY-CHAIN GENE is assembled from four sets of sequences in the germ-line configuration (*top*): *L/V*, *D*, *J* and *C*. Somatic recombination brings together one of the *L/V* sequences, a *D* and a *J* to code for the variable region of the chain. As in the case of the light-chain gene, the constant-region DNA (*C*) is downstream, separated by a noncoding sequence. In the heavy chain, however, there are eight separate *C* sequences, each one coding for a different constant region. (Each *C* sequence is divided into from three to five domains, but sequences are diagrammed in simplified form.) Final assembly of coding sequences is accomplished by RNA processing.

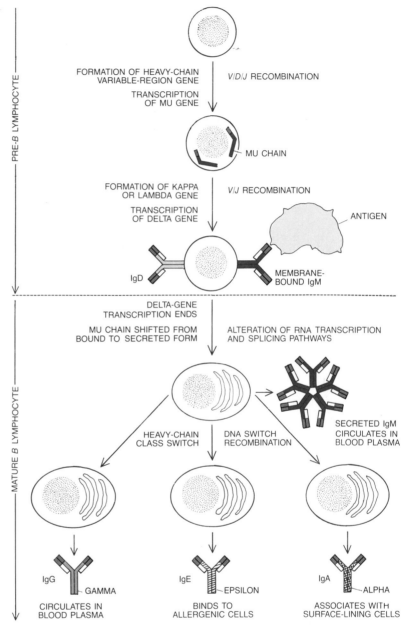

Figure 2.8 DIFFERENTIATION of antibody-producing cells is traced beginning with the pre-*B* lymphocyte. At each stage the major genetic events are listed (*left*), along with the pertinent gene-shuffling mechanisms (*right*). The heavy chain is manufactured first, then the light chain (kappa or lambda). IgM and IgD are displayed on the cell surface. When a specific antigen is recognized and bound by a surface antibody, the cell is driven further in development: it proliferates to form a clone of mature *B* lymphocytes, which are specialized to synthesize large amounts of protein. Now the expression and the arrangement of the heavy-chain constant-region gene may change, so that different types of antibody are produced.

specific variable region (a product of *V/D/J* recombination). This heavy chain at first remains inside the pre-*B* cell. Then, after the onset of light-chain and delta heavy-chain synthesis, both the mu and the delta heavy chains combine with the light chains to form complete IgM and IgD molecules.

The next stage in development is distinguished by the concurrent appearance of both IgM and IgD on the cell surface. Both antibodies have the same variable region and so both are directed against the same antigen.

The subsequent steps in lymphocyte maturation

are apparently antigen-driven. The primary event of the immune process is called clonal selection. An antigen binds to a receptor: the best-fitting antigen-combining site among millions or billions of surface immunoglobulins. By this interaction the cell displaying the selected immunoglobulin is driven farther along its developmental pathway. It proliferates to form a clone of antibody-producing B lymphocytes.

In the course of B-cell maturation the IgD and IgM disappear from the cell surface and either IgM, IgG, IgE or IgA is instead secreted by the cell. Each of these classes of immunoglobulins has a different heavy-chain constant region, but antibodies of any class that are synthesized in a given cell have the same variable regions, namely the ones that were assembled in the precursor cell and that formed the combining site selected by the antigen. Because each heavy chain gives the antibody a different effector function, the same variable region can take part in different immune reactions. The process by which the same variable region appears in association with different heavy-chain constant regions is called heavy-chain class switching. The lymphocyte depends on two mechanisms to carry out class switching. One mechanism is based on differential RNA transcription and splicing, the other on a version of DNA recombination.

The arrangement of the heavy-chain genes in mouse embryonic DNA, extending over more than 100,000 nucleotides, has been deciphered by several groups of investigators in the past three years. Hood and Tonegawa and their co-workers contributed principally to understanding of the structure of the mu, gamma and alpha genes. Frederick R. Blattner and his associates at the University of Wisconsin at Madison established the location of the delta gene. Tasuku Honjo and his associates in the Osaka University Faculty of Medicine were able to clone and map the gamma genes (there are four IgG subclasses) and link them to one another and in turn to the epsilon and alpha genes. The arrangement of these genes (reading from upstream to downstream, or from the 5′ end to the 3′ end of the sequence) is mu, delta, gamma 3, gamma 1, gamma 2b, gamma 2a, epsilon and alpha.

BOUND AND SECRETED IgM

How is it that IgM can appear successively in two forms, one bound to the lymphocyte membrane and the other secreted? Jonathan W. Uhr of the University of Texas Health Science Center at Dallas first noted a structural difference between the membrane-bound mu chain and the secreted one. More detailed studies indicate that the membrane-bound form ends in a short sequence of hydrophobic amino acids, which evidently anchor the antibody in the cell's membrane through their affinity for the hydrophobic lipids of the membrane. The secreted mu chain lacks the hydrophobic sequence. Hood, with Randall Wall of the University of California at Los Angeles, and Baltimore and his co-workers at MIT showed that two forms of messenger RNA are synthesized from the mu gene. In one form the message stops just short of two small coding segments that specify the anchor sequence; in the other form the segments coding for the anchor sequence are included.

Each heavy-chain constant region is encoded in from three to six separate coding domains separated by short intervening sequences of noninformational DNA. As in the case of most other split genes, the primary transcript of the heavy-chain genes includes both the coding sequences and the intervening sequences. RNA processing thereupon splices the coding sequences to one another, eliminating the noninformational segments. The primary transcript of the mu gene sometimes includes the coding sequence for the hydrophobic anchor; if it is present, the enzymes that process the RNA splice it to the end of the main mu messenger so as to exclude a "stop" codon that would otherwise halt translation at the end of the main message. If the primary RNA transcript lacks the anchor sequence, no splicing takes place; the stop codon preceding the anchor sequence is recognized and the secretable form of the mu chain is synthesized (see Figure 2.9). There is increasing evidence that many of the other heavy chains, and perhaps all of them, have a similar arrangement allowing them either to be anchored to the membrane or to be secreted.

The simultaneous appearance of mu and delta chains is likely to be due to similar splicing alternatives. Transcription proceeds through the variable-region DNA and then through the several domains of the mu gene. A certain fraction of the primary transcripts end in a way that yields mu chains, as described above. Another fraction of the transcripts continue for a few thousand nucleotides and therefore include not only the V/D/J and mu sequences but also the delta sequence. Among the many options for splicing such transcripts, one is to splice the V/D/J DNA directly to the beginning of the delta-gene transcript. In this way two messenger RNA's are formed simultaneously; one specifies the mu

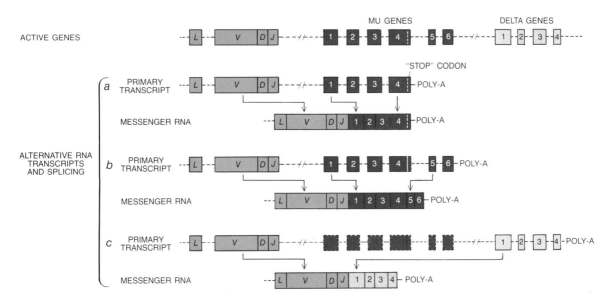

Figure 2.9 RNA TRANSCRIPTION of the heavy-chain genes for the variable region and for the mu and delta constant regions in an antibody-producing cell. If transcription ends at the fourth coding domain of the mu gene (*a*), the RNA is spliced to yield a coherent messenger RNA for a chain lacking a short amino acid sequence that would anchor the chain to the cell wall; IgM is secreted. If the transcript includes mu domains 5 and 6 (*b*), splicing removes the "stop" codon and brings the last two domains, encoding the anchor sequence, into the messenger RNA; the IgM is membrane-bound. If the primary transcript includes the delta gene (*c*), splicing sometimes eliminates the mu gene and connects the delta domains directly to *J* making IgD.

heavy chain and one the delta chain, but both encode the same variable region. Translation of the two RNA's into protein leads to the simultaneous display on the cell surface of IgM and IgD that have the same antigen specificity.

A second mechanism that shuffles heavy-chain genes depends on the rearrangement of DNA sequences to accomplish the remaining steps of the heavy-chain class switch (see Figure 2.10). In contrast to the rather precise nature of the *V/J* and *V/J/D* joining events, the recombination process that leads to the expression of a particular heavy-chain class has a much greater degree of freedom.

Consider the switch from the mu chain to the alpha chain (from IgM to IgA). The active heavy-chain gene is arranged so that the variable-region coding sequence is a long way—about 8,000 nucleotides—from the first constant-region coding sequence (namely the first mu sequence). Ordinarily this noncoding spacer region is excised from the primary RNA transcript for the mu chain. Although the spacer region has no known coding function, it does have a stretch of about 2,000 nucleotides that, both Hood and Tonegawa and their co-workers

showed, includes a series of repeated nucleotide sequences of various sizes.

In our laboratory Ravetch and Ilan R. Kirsch were able to show that the 2,000-nucleotide segment with the repeated blocks is similar in sequence to a stretch of DNA far downstream, adjacent to the alpha gene. Switching from IgM to IgA must involve recombination of these distant similar sequences; they apparently serve as switch signals to join the *V/D/J* sequence to the alpha coding sequence, deleting mu and the other constant-region genes. Since there are no coding sequences within the switch regions, the exact crossover points in the recombination event can apparently vary widely within the region. Both Tonegawa and Honjo have found analogous switch regions adjacent to the gamma genes. They have suggested that these regions constitute a signal for the switch from mu to gamma.

BROAD IMPLICATIONS

Not many years ago geneticists and molecular biologists had come to accept as axiomatic the principles

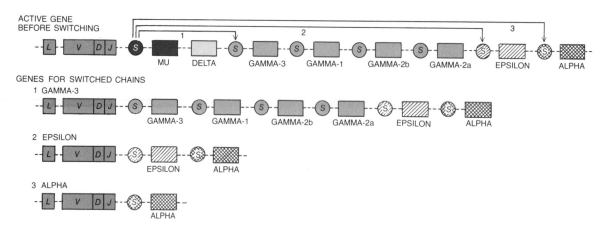

Figure 2.10 HEAVY-CHAIN CLASS SWITCH is accomplished by DNA recombination. As long as a lymphocyte is synthesizing mu or delta chains the heavy-chain gene is arranged as is shown at the top. Each constant-region gene is preceded by a switching signal (S) having some complementary relation to a similar signal between the variable-region sequences and the mu gene. The signals apparently mediate a recombination that joins a $V/D/J$ sequence to one of the downstream constant-region sequences; three such possibilities are shown. The switched DNA is transcribed and the RNA is spliced to make a messenger RNA encoding the gamma-3, the epsilon or the alpha region.

that every protein chain is encoded by a particular germ-line gene, that the total genome present in embryonic cells remains unchanged as somatic cells differentiate to form various tissues and that the distinctive shapes and functions of the differentiated cells lie in the differential expression of the same genes. The discovery that the immune system generates many millions or billions of proteins by shuffling a few hundred germ-line genes shows that the principles do not always hold true. Proteins other than antibodies may also require more information than can readily be provided by an unaltered linear genome, and so it seems likely that somatic DNA recombination and selective RNA transcription and splicing may also operate to provide diversity in cells other than lymphocytes.

One indication that such mechanisms may be applied outside the immune system comes from an experiment done recently in my laboratory by Kirsch, Ravetch, Max and Robert L. Ney. They used the mu-alpha switch as a probe with which to search for any similar stretches of DNA in the mouse and the human genomes. Each probe identified from 10 to 15 fragments of DNA able to hybridize with the recombination signals. This seemed far too many to be accounted for by the need for

heavy-chain class switching. The probe was then applied to the DNA of lymphocytes in which all heavy-chain genes between the V genes and the last constant-region gene, on both chromosomes, had been deleted. Again the probe recognized some 10 or 15 fragments, demonstrating that the "extra" signals are encoded outside the constant-region sequences, that is, elsewhere in the organism's genetic apparatus.

The implication is that such switching signals mediate the somatic recombination of other genes, for other proteins requiring a high degree of diversity. For example, recombination might serve to generate the diverse protein "addresses" that appear on the surface of embryonic cells and seem to guide them to a specific place and destiny in a complex organism. Or it might help to generate the diverse population of antigen receptors on the surface of T cells, a class of regulatory lymphocytes. Such possibilities remain to be investigated. What is clear is that the immune system has demonstrated the enormous potential of gene shuffling, which greatly increases the genetic information available for making antibodies and is likely to be central to the development of diversity in other gene systems as well.

The *T* Cell and Its Receptor

The T *cell plays a key role in the body's capacity to fight viral infection, but it also acts to reject grafted tissue. Experiments have now identified the molecule that underlies this behavior.*

· · ·

Philippa Marrack and John Kappler
February, 1986

The cells of the immune system are responsible for the ability of vertebrate animals to recognize that antigens, or foreign materials, have invaded their bodies. The immune response that follows is remarkable for its specificity. A person immunized by vaccination against smallpox, for example, can resist infection by the smallpox virus but not by, say, the influenza virus. In the past decade immunologists have come to recognize that the most important factor in the ability of the immune system to react specifically to viruses is a class of small cells called *T* lymphocytes, or *T* cells. The *T* cells also play an essential auxiliary role in the immune response to bacterial infection.

It has long been accepted that the trigger for this activity is a molecule embedded in the membrane of the *T* cell called the *T*-cell receptor. A specific antigen is assumed to fit and bind to the receptor as a key fits into a lock, thereby setting in motion the complex series of biochemical events that constitute the immune response. For a variety of reasons the isolation of the *T*-cell receptor has proved to be exceedingly difficult, and until quite recently its properties have had to be inferred indirectly, without the guidance afforded by a knowledge of its structure. That structure is now rapidly coming into focus.

The structural clarification of the *T*-cell receptor is bringing about a far better understanding of the complex interactions of *T* cells with other elements of the immune system. In particular, it is becoming apparent that the *T* cell is specially suited for dealing with infections associated with the cells of the host, rather than with infections that circulate freely in the host's bodily fluids. To carry out this role the *T*-cell receptor must not only recognize a specific antigen but also recognize certain membrane proteins of the host cell itself. Such a recognition mechanism must be kept under tight control, for if a *T* cell were to be activated by the host proteins alone, it could readily turn against the healthy cells of the organism. The consequent delicacy of the *T* cell's recognition system leads to its many fascinating and medically important properties. For example, *T* cells will rapidly act to reject foreign tissue that is surgically grafted or transplanted into the body. Hence the investigation of the *T*-cell receptor is an issue of major interest to surgery.

There are actually two kinds of lymphocyte responsible for the recognition of specific antigens: the second kind is the *B* cell. Both the *B* cell and the *T* cell are derived from the bone marrow, but the *T* cell undergoes further development in the thymus gland, just under the upper part of the breastbone in man. Both *B* and *T* cells circulate in the blood and the lymph and are concentrated in the major lymphatic organs: the lymph nodes and the spleen in higher vertebrates. They can be quite long-lived; in man they can persist for many years without dividing. In response to an antigen, however, lymphocytes enlarge considerably, divide rapidly and secrete a number of protein factors that contribute to the elimination of the invading organism or foreign material.

It has been known for some time that the initial response of the *B* cell to an antigen is mediated by a receptor protein displayed on the cell membrane. The antigen binds to the receptor, and the binding leads the *B* cell to divide and differentiate into a clone of plasma cells. These cells secrete antibodies that have the same antigen-binding properties as the receptor molecules embedded in the surface of the parent *B* cell. Indeed, the antibody is identical with the *B*-cell receptor to which the antigen was originally bound, except that the end of the chain of amino acids anchoring the receptor protein in the membrane of the *B* cell is not found on the soluble antibody. Both *B*-cell receptors and antibodies are also called immunoglobulins.

Once the antibodies are secreted into the blood or the lymph, they bind to free antigen and mark it for destruction by other components of the immune system. This general picture of how a *B* cell is "selected" by an antigen for the capacity of the cell to clonally expand and secrete antibody to the antigen is called the clonal-selection theory; it was developed in the 1960's by Sir Macfarlane Burnet of the Walter and Eliza Hall Institute for Medical Research in Melbourne, David W. Talmage, then at the University of Chicago, and Niels Kaj Jerne, then at the World Health Organization.

In their role as *B*-cell receptors the antibodies are found in quite small quantities. When the *B* cell is challenged with antigen, however, the antibodies appear in serum in large and soluble quantities. Antibodies are also secreted at high levels by certain types of *B*-cell tumor such as plasmacytomas. The ready availability of such high concentrations of soluble antibody and the fact that each antibody molecule can bind to antigen made it possible to isolate antibodies relatively easily and learn a great deal about the structure of the *B*-cell receptor.

The *T*-cell receptor has been much more elusive. The *T* cell, like the *B* cell, responds to an antigen by clonally dividing and differentiating into one of several kinds of *T* cell specific to the antigen. Cytotoxic *T* cells bind to viral antigen displayed on the surface of an infected cell and kill the cell. Suppressor *T* cells act to inhibit the immune response to an antigen some time after the response has been set in motion. Helper *T* cells bind to antigen on the surface of a *B* cell that has already bound itself to the antigen. Each helper *T* cell then releases hormone-like molecules called lymphokines that enable the *B* cell to multiply and differentiate. Thus there is a two-key system for releasing the enormous destructive potential of a *B* cell: one key (the free antigen) for the *B*-cell receptor and the other key (the antigen on the surface of the *B* cell) for the *T*-cell receptor.

T cells themselves never differentiate into cells that secrete antibodies. Hence unlike the *B*-cell receptor, the *T*-cell receptor is not readily available in the quantities of purified, soluble chemical that are needed for convenient analysis. Because antibodies are so elegantly constructed and so efficient in their capacity to recognize antigens, it was assumed for many years that the *T* cell would rely on the same molecules as the *B* cell does in order to bind and respond to antigen.

Many investigators spent years examining the surfaces of *T* cells and their secretions for immunoglobulins. Although extensive searches have suggested that suppressor *T* cells may bind antigen with molecules similar to immunoglobulin, many experiments have shown that most *T* cells are not associated with immunoglobulins. Not only are immunoglobulins not secreted by *T* cells but also they are not found either on the membranes of *T* cells or in their cytoplasm. Other experiments show that *T* cells do not express messenger RNA transcribed from immunoglobulin genes; moreover, when one examines the immunoglobulin genes in the *T* cell, one finds that the *T* cell does not usually rearrange them the way the *B* cell does.

Such negative results accumulated in the 1970's and in the early 1980's. Although the results of such experiments are not usually very persuasive when they are considered one at a time, the sheer number of failures gradually led molecular immunologists to change their approach. If immunoglobulins could not be found in association with *T* cells, one would have to look elsewhere for the *T*-cell receptor for antigen.

The study of foreign tissue grafts and their rejection by a host animal had led cellular immunologists to the same conclusion some years earlier. For example, mouse cells taken from one strain of mice are rejected rapidly after being injected into a mouse of a different genetic strain. Beginning in the early 1930's Peter Gorer and other workers showed that such rejection is caused by antigenic molecules on the surfaces of the foreign mouse cells.

The proteins that mark every cell as "foreign" or "self" are encoded by genes linked close together in a region of DNA called the major histocompatibility complex (MHC), after the prefix "histo-," meaning tissue. The proteins themselves are called MHC-encoded proteins. One of their most remarkable properties is their extreme polymorphism: there are many alleles, or variants, for the MHC genes encoding each protein. Hence the likelihood that two unrelated individuals have identical MHC-encoded proteins is small.

Following the work of Gorer it became increasingly clear that graft rejection and the MHC-encoded proteins are closely related to the immune response. Sir Peter Medawar and others demonstrated that lymphocytes are responsible for recognizing the antigenic molecules on a graft of foreign tissue; later work showed that the lymphocytes central to the graft rejection are *T* cells rather than *B* cells. Graft transplantation is not an experiment of nature, however, and so immunologists were still in doubt about the functions of the MHC-encoded proteins.

Some clues about such functions began to emerge in the mid-1960's. Hugh O. McDevitt, then at the National Institute for Medical Research in England, Michael Sela of the Weizmann Institute of Science in Israel and Baruj Benacerraf, then at New York University School of Medicine, and his colleagues studied the response of various strains of animals to antigens. They found that the response of a mouse to certain synthetic antigens can depend on the genetic strain of the mouse. For example, when the polymer known as TGAL is injected into mice, the mice bearing *b* alleles in their MHC make antibodies to the polymer, but the mice bearing *k* alleles in their MHC do not. It soon became apparent that these genes act by affecting the functions of *T* cells and not some other cell type in the immune system.

Some immunologists then suggested the *T*-cell receptor might be encoded by the MHC. If it were, one would naturally expect different kinds of MHC to encode different *T*-cell receptors, and the latter would account for differences in the response to TGAL from one mouse strain to another. The theory had to be discarded when it was discovered that some of the MHC-encoded proteins that affect the binding of TGAL are not even expressed on the surface of the *T* cell in mice. Hence the source of

the observed differences could not be the *T*-cell receptor alone, and there was no further point in supposing the receptor was encoded by the MHC. The experiment did lend support to a subtler point: the differences in the antibody response to TGAL indicated that MHC-encoded proteins affect the way TGAL is recognized by the *T*-cell receptor. This finding was the first clue that some interaction between foreign antigens and MHC-encoded proteins was a prerequisite for the action of the receptor.

How could one account for such a strange collection of results? The answers came from the pioneering work of Ethan M. Shevach and Alan S. Rosenthal at the National Institute of Allergy and Infectious Diseases, David H. Katz and Benacerraf at the Harvard Medical School, Bernice Kindred at the University of Constance in West Germany, Donald Shreffler of the University of Michigan School of Medicine and, most clearly, from the remarkable experiments of Rolf Zinkernagel and Peter C. Doherty of the Australian National University.

In one experiment Zinkernagel and Doherty injected sublethal doses of a virus known as LCM (for lymphocytic choriomeningitis) into mice and isolated LCM-specific, cytotoxic *T* cells from the immunized animals (see Figure 3.1). The usual function of such *T* cells is to recognize viral antigens on infected cells and destroy the cells. Most strains of mice make antibodies to LCM virus, and so there was little chance that LCM virus would fail to induce an immune response in some strains of mice the way TGAL does. Nevertheless, Zinkernagel and Doherty found to their surprise that the *T* cells from *k*-strain, LCM-immunized mice are able to kill cells infected with the LCM virus only if the infected cells bear at least one of several kinds of *k*-strain, MHC-encoded proteins. In other words, the *T* cells that were lethal to infected cells bearing certain *k*-strain, MHC-encoded proteins could not kill cells from closely related mice, infected with the same virus but bearing, say, the *d* strain of the same MHC-encoded proteins.

This experiment and others demonstrated that cytotoxic *T* cells were paying attention not only to viral antigens on the infected cell but also to the amino acid sequences of MHC-encoded proteins on the same infected cell. Other investigators quickly showed that the same was true for cytotoxic *T* cells specific for other antigens. The phenomenon is now called MHC restriction. In general the MHC-encoded proteins recognized by the cytotoxic *T* cells

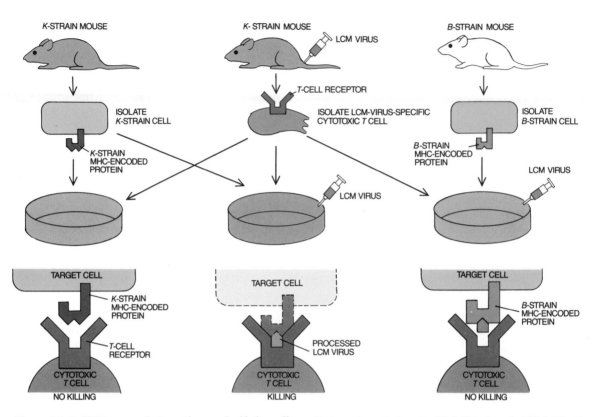

Figure 3.1 *T* CELL responds to antigen only if the cell binds both the antigen and an MHC-encoded protein on the target cell. *T* cells taken from a *k*-strain mouse immunized with lymphocytic choriomeningitis (LCM) virus can kill cells bearing *k*-strain, MHC-encoded proteins after the cells have been infected with LCM virus (*middle*). The *T* cells cannot kill cells infected with the virus that do not bear the *k*-strain, MHC-encoded proteins (*right*), and of course they do not kill uninfected mouse cells that bear the *k*-strain proteins (*left*).

belong to a single structural class called the class I proteins; they are found on the surfaces of all nucleated cells in the body.

We and several other investigators then found that helper *T* cells are also MHC-restricted; in general, however, the helper *T* cell recognizes a different class of MHC-encoded proteins called the class II proteins. The expression of class II proteins is considerably less widespread in the body than the expression of class I proteins: in people the class II proteins are found only on *T* cells, *B* cells, macrophages and certain cells of other tissues.

As soon as MHC restriction was discovered it was clear that two kinds of theory could account for the facts. One, the associated-recognition theory, suggests in its extremest form that each *T* cell bears receptors of a single kind. Each such receptor would somehow bind a complex of the antigen and a particular MHC-encoded protein that appear on the surface of the antigen-presenting cell. The second theory, which is called the dual-recognition theory, suggests in its extremest form that each *T* cell bears two kinds of receptor: one would bind a specific antigen and the other would bind a specific MHC-encoded protein.

There are advantages and disadvantages to each kind of theory. The associated-recognition theory accounts for the observation that *T* cells only rarely bind to antigen or to MHC-encoded proteins without binding to both molecules at the same time. Moreover, the theory accounts nicely for the findings of McDevitt, Sela and Benacerraf on the immunogenic properties of TGAL in mice. If a single

T-cell receptor must simultaneously bind a complex of antigen and MHC-encoded protein, the failure of *k*-strain mice to respond to TGAL might be caused by the failure of the TGAL antigen to form a complex with the *k*-strain, MHC-encoded protein. On the other hand, the dual-recognition theory does not share a disadvantage of the associated-recognition theory: it need not postulate an interaction between every form of antigen and the invariant forms of MHC-encoded protein that are found in any individual animal.

Although the final word is not yet in, it is probably fair to say that the current data favor the associated-recognition theory, with its model of a single *T*-cell receptor for antigen and MHC-encoded protein. For example, we have studied the properties of hybrid T cells that express *T*-cell receptors inherited from two different parents (see Figure 3.2). We first isolated helper *T* cells that specifically recognize an antigen, chicken ovalbumin (cOVA), when it is associated with certain *k*-strain, class II proteins. We fused the *T* cells to a T-cell tumor in order to make a *T*-cell hybridoma, a hybrid cell that grows rapidly and clones readily in tissue culture.

In order to construct a cell having two different sets of *T*-cell receptors we fused one of our *T*-cell-hybridoma cells with a second set of antigen-specific *T* cells. The second set of *T* cells could respond only to the keyhole-limpet hemocyanin (KLH) antigen in the presence of *f*-strain, class II proteins.

We tested the response of the newly fused *T* cells to cOVA or KLH antigens in association with *k*-strain or *f*-strain antigen-presenting cells. If the dual-recognition theory were correct, one would expect that the newly fused *T* cells would bear four types of receptor, one for each antigen and one for each class II, MHC-encoded protein. Hence they would respond to both antigens presented on a *k*-strain cell and to both antigens presented on an *f*-strain cell. Instead we found they would respond to the antigens only as their parents did: to cOVA associated with *k*-strain cells and to KLH associated with *f*-strain cells. There was no sign of a response to cOVA on *f*-strain cells or to KLH on *k*-strain cells.

If the associated-recognition theory is correct, the antigen and the MHC-encoded protein must somehow form a complex before a *T* cell can bind to them. The results of several experiments suggest there is some kind of interaction between MHC-encoded proteins and antigens, but only a few experiments have been able to detect the interaction directly. Perhaps the most striking recent demonstration of such an interaction comes from the work of Emil R. Unanue and his colleagues at Washington University School of Medicine.

Unanue and his colleagues identified a small antigen that can be recognized by *T* cells when it is associated with *k*-strain, MHC-encoded proteins but not when it is associated with *d*-strain proteins. They placed equal concentrations of the antigen in solution on both sides of a semipermeable membrane, and they placed one or the other strain of MHC-encoded proteins on one side of the membrane. Because the antigen molecule is significantly smaller than either kind of protein, the membrane allowed free passage of the antigens but restricted the proteins to their initial compartment.

Unanue and his group found that when *k*-strain, MHC-encoded proteins were added to one compartment and the antigen concentration was allowed to equilibrate, the concentration of the antigen became higher in the compartment holding the *k*-strain proteins. The concentrations of the antigen in the two compartments did not change when the *d*-strain, MHC-encoded proteins were added to one compartment. The result suggests that antigen does bind, at least sometimes, to the MHC-encoded protein with which it is recognized, although the process may not take place very efficiently.

Even after all the foregoing properties of the *T*-cell receptor had been established, the identity of the protein responsible for its activity was still a mystery. It was clear by then, however, that the *T*-cell receptor differs in at least one important way from the antibody molecule. Whether the *T*-cell receptor is one distinct protein or two, at least some component of the receptor has a strong tendency to recognize part of an MHC-encoded protein. The antibody molecule does not.

There were two major technological breakthroughs that enabled investigators to begin to discern the structure of the *T*-cell receptor. One was a discovery made in the early 1970's by George Köhler and Cesar Milstein at the Medical Research Council's Laboratory of Molecular Biology in Cambridge; the two workers found a way to produce B-cell hybridomas that can secrete large quantities of selected kinds of antibody in vitro. Such antibodies are called monoclonal antibodies, and they can be produced and purified in enormous quantities. The second breakthrough was the development of methods whereby *T*-cell clones or *T*-cell hybrid-

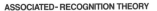

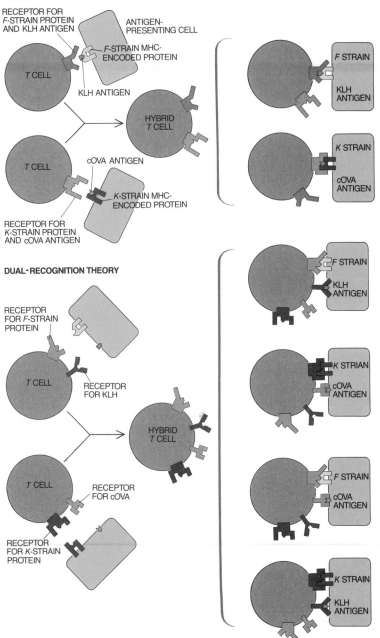

Figure 3.2 ASSOCIATED-RECOGNI-TION THEORY asserts that each *T* cell bears a single receptor, which can bind a combination of antigen and MHC-encoded protein (*upper left*). The dual-recognition theory asserts that each (*T*) cell bears two different receptors, one receptor for antigen and one for the MHC-encoded protein (*lower left*). The authors constructed a hybrid (*T*) cell by fusing two normal (*T*) cells. One parent (*T*) cell was isolated from animals having *f*-strain, MHC-encoded proteins, after the animals were immunized against the antigen keyhole-limpet hemocyanin (KLH). The second parent *T* cell was isolated from *k*-strain animals immunized against the antigen chicken ovalbumin (cOVA).

omas for specific antigens and specific MHC-encoded proteins could be propagated in culture. We and a number of other investigators have exploited both breakthroughs to create antibodies to *T*-cell receptors and thereby identify structural properties of the *T*-cell receptor.

To make antibodies to a *T*-cell receptor we first built a *T*-cell hybridoma that bore a receptor for recognizing cOVA antigen in association with a *d*-strain, class II protein. When the receptors on such hybridomas are engaged with the right antigen and the right MHC-encoded protein, they respond rapidly by secreting lymphokines. Such hybridomas are convenient experimentally because the production of lymphokines can be induced and quickly measured in culture.

To make an antibody of known specificity one must immunize an animal against a known antigen, but in the case of the *T*-cell receptor the precise identity of the antigen was not known. Our strategy was to immunize mice against the *T*-cell hybridomas, in the hope of inducing the production of antibodies that would interfere only with functions presumably carried out by the receptors on the hybridomas. We reasoned that an antibody to the receptor would bind to the receptor and block its ability to engage cOVA and *d*-strain, MHC-encoded protein. A decrease in the production of lymphokines would indicate the blockage.

We immunized many mice against large numbers of *T*-cell hybridomas. We then drew serum from each mouse at various times after the immunizations and tested the serums in culture for their ability to block the response of the *T*-cell hybridomas to *d*-strain cells and cOVA. Eventually we identified several mice that made the blocking antibody. The antiserums of these mice had an additional encouraging property: when *T*-cell hybridomas of a different specificity were challenged in culture with the antigen and MHC-encoded protein to which they were specific, the mouse antiserums did not block the *T*-cell response. We repeated the experiment with other *T*-cell hybridomas in the role of the original hybridoma. In each case the blocking antibodies developed by the mice were effective only against the *T*-cell hybridoma used for the immunization.

The specificity of such antiserums for a particular *T*-cell hybridoma led us to believe we had indeed produced antibodies to a particular *T*-cell receptor. The *T*-cell receptor is the only structure on the surface of the *T*-cell hybridoma that one would expect to be blocked by an antibody in such a specific way, because it alone should vary from one *T*-cell clone to another. Nevertheless, our task was not yet finished. Because only small amounts of the antibodies could be isolated from each mouse, we applied the method of Köhler and Milstein to immortalize the antibody-secreting cells.

Kathryn Haskins and Janice White of our laboratory extracted plasma *B* cells from one of the mice immune to the cOVA *T*-cell hybridoma. The plasma cells were fused with tumor cells to make plasma-cell hybridomas that would readily grow in culture. The plasma-cell hybridomas secreted antibodies, which were then screened for their ability to block the recognition of cOVA and *d*-strain, class II protein by the cOVA *T*-cell hybridoma. One plasma-cell hybridoma had this property. Similar antibodies were obtained at about the same time by James P. Allison, then at the University of Texas Cancer Center in Smithville, Tex., and by Stefan C. W. Meuer and Ellis Reinherz of the Harvard Medical School.

It is primarily the successful preparation of antibodies for specific *T*-cell receptors that has made it possible to build up a picture of the *T*-cell-receptor protein. The tight bond between the receptor and the antibody has enabled investigators to purify the receptor in large enough quantities to reveal its basic molecular properties. Perhaps surprisingly, it turns out there is a close structural resemblance between the antibody molecule and the *T*-cell receptor. Both are made up of two polypeptide chains encoded by distinct genes in the DNA and held together by strong, covalent bonds connecting two sulfur atoms (see Figure 3.3). In antibodies the two chains differ in size; they are called the heavy chain and the light chain. Each chain includes a sequence of amino acids that is relatively constant within an animal, even for antibodies that bind to distinct antigens. In addition each chain has a long stretch of amino acids that varies considerably for antibodies of different antigen specificity.

The variability of antibody within an animal arises from the genome. The basic idea is that each polypeptide chain of the antibody is made up of three or four regions, each of which can be encoded by one of several randomly selected pieces of DNA. The combinatorial variability arising from the construction leads to a large number of distinct antibodies.

For example, a heavy chain is made up of four

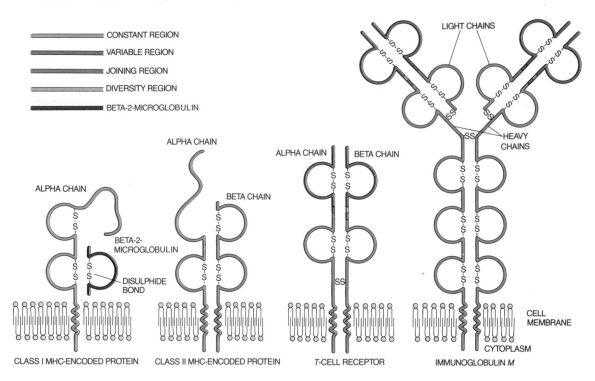

CONSTANT REGION
VARIABLE REGION
JOINING REGION
DIVERSITY REGION
BETA-2-MICROGLOBULIN

ALPHA CHAIN

ALPHA CHAIN

ALPHA CHAIN

BETA CHAIN

LIGHT CHAINS

BETA-2-
MICROGLOBULIN

BETA CHAIN

HEAVY
CHAINS

ALPHA CHAIN

DISULPHIDE
BOND

CELL
MEMBRANE

CYTOPLASM

CLASS I MHC-ENCODED PROTEIN

CLASS II MHC-ENCODED PROTEIN

T-CELL RECEPTOR

IMMUNOGLOBULIN M

Figure 3.3 MOLECULAR STRUCTURES of the class I MHC-encoded protein, the class II protein, the T-cell receptor and the immunoglobulin, or antibody, molecule are similar, and the molecules also share similar sequences of amino acids. The molecules are characterized by loops made up of about 70 amino acids within each chain; sulfur atoms at each end of the loop are joined by covalent bonds.

Class I proteins are expressed on the surface of every nucleated cell in higher vertebrates, in association with the non-MHC-encoded protein beta-2-microglobulin. Class II proteins are expressed only on the surface of selected cells. Variable, joining and diversity regions have been identified in the T-cell receptor and in the immunoglobulin.

regions of amino acids: the constant region, a joining region, a diversity region and the variable region. The constant region is encoded by only one piece of DNA, but the strand of DNA coding for the joining region can be drawn at random from one of four distinct segments. Similarly, the diversity region is encoded by one of more than 10 pieces of DNA and the variable region is encoded by one of more than 100. The total number of different amino acid sequences that can arise from the different combinations is thus more than $4 \times 10 \times 100$, or 4,000. The light chain is also made up of different combinations of DNA, and additional variability arises because of imprecise points of contact between the joining, diversity and variable regions. According to Susumu Tonegawa of the Massachusetts Institute of Technology, the number of distinct antibody molecules may be as great as one billion [see "The Molecules of the Immune System," by Susumu Tonegawa; SCIENTIFIC AMERICAN, October, 1985].

In the T-cell receptor the two chains are called the alpha chain and the beta chain. In the mouse both have a molecular weight of about 43,000 atomic mass units (a.m.u.); in people the alpha chain weighs about 50,000 a.m.u. and the beta chain weighs about 39,000. By comparing the alpha chains and the beta chains from different T-cell clones with one another we found that certain fixed sequences of amino acids appear on each chain from clone to clone. Other sequences can vary from clone to clone.

With the discovery of the proteins that make up the T-cell receptor, the techniques of molecular biology could be called into play. Such techniques enable workers to analyze the genes that encode a protein of interest, and that analysis can disclose the structure of a protein much faster than biochemical methods can. Moreover, given the similar roles of *T*-cell receptors and immunoglobulins in the immune system and the emerging structural similarities between them, it seemed likely that the segments of DNA encoding the *T*-cell receptor would be rearranged before its constituent proteins are expressed on the surface of the *T* cell, much as the segments of DNA encoding the *B*-cell receptor are. The race was soon on to find the *T*-cell receptor genes.

The first serious candidates for the genes were reported simultaneously by two groups: Stephen M. Hedrick, Mark M. Davis and their collaborators at the National Institutes of Health, the University of California at San Diego and Stanford University, and Tak W. Mak and his group at the Ontario Cancer Institute. Both groups, the first group working with mouse genes and the second working with human genes, reasoned that *T*-cell-receptor proteins would be found only in *T* cells and not, for example, in *B* cells. They adopted elegant experimental techniques to exploit this assumption, and they were soon able to identify genes expressed only in *B* cells or only in *T* cells but not in both kinds of lymphocyte. The genes encoding the beta chain of the receptor were identified first, and within another year the genes for the alpha chain were isolated as well. Much detail about the structure of the *T*-cell receptor has been derived from the analysis of these genes.

Both the alpha and the beta chain of the *T*-cell receptor have variable, constant and joining regions. In addition investigators have confirmed a diversity region in the beta chain, and the alpha chain may have one too. The amino acid sequences of each of these regions are similar to their analogues in the immunoglobulins, but they are by no means identical.

Davis and his collaborators and Leroy Hood and his colleagues at the California Institute of Technology have studied the organization of the DNA sequences that encode the beta chain. So far they have found 12 joining regions, two diversity regions (each of which can be read in any one of three transcription frames) and about 20 variable regions. The number of possible amino acid combinations in the beta chain is therefore at least $12 \times 2 \times 3 \times 20$, or 1,440. Even that number is much too small: a realistic estimate of the variability must also take account of mutations and imprecise joining, which affect the *T*-cell receptor just as they affect the anti-

body molecule. The variability in the alpha chain may be even greater: although no diversity regions have yet been identified, there appear to be many more joining and variable regions than there are for the beta chain — perhaps as many as 100 of each kind. The alpha and beta chains can therefore combine to form on the order of 10 million different kinds of *T*-cell receptor, which is enough to account for the known repertoire of *T* cells in an animal.

The new structural information on the *T*-cell receptor makes it possible to recast many of the traditional questions about the immune system in much sharper terms. There are essentially three kinds of observed recognition event for which one would now like to give a structural account. First, the *T*-cell does not respond to the MHC-encoded proteins of the self, or in other words it tolerates the self. Second, the *T* cell responds when it is confronted simultaneously with an antigen and a self-MHC-encoded protein, but usually not when it is confronted with an antigen in association with an MHC-encoded protein of another strain of animal. Third, the *T* cell also responds to an MHC-encoded protein from another individual in the absence of antigen; it is this effect that accounts for the rejection of grafted or transplanted tissue. There is a developmental question associated with these observations: How do precursor *T* cells become differentiated in the thymus into cells that have such properties?

The most straightforward explanation for tolerance is that *T*-cell clones reacting to self-MHC-encoded proteins are somehow eliminated in the thymus. There is not yet any clear account of how the screening might take place. One suggestion is that at some stage in their development *T* cells die if their antigen-specific receptors bind any molecule expressed by the cells of the organism. This idea is known as the clonal-abortion theory; it asserts that as *T* cells develop, all *T* cells that react specifically to self-MHC-encoded proteins or to other self antigens would be killed because they are continuously bombarded by such molecules. *T* cells reacting specifically to self-MHC-encoded proteins associated with foreign antigen would also die if they were to bind such complexes, but in an uninfected animal such *T* cells would develop to full maturity. They could then survive until an invading foreign antigen triggered their response.

The response of the *T* cell to an MHC-encoded protein associated with an antigen raises its own

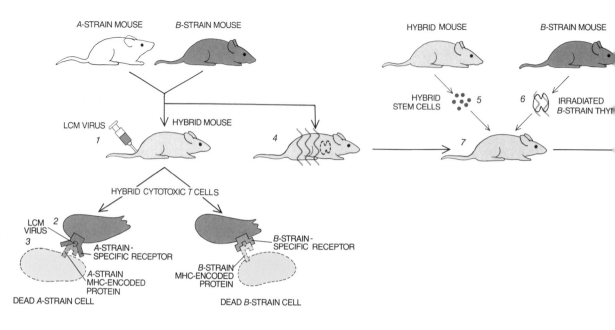

puzzles. Rolf Zinkernagel and his colleagues and Michael J. Bevan, then at MIT, first recognized the dimensions of the problem in their study of the "education" of the T cells in the thymus (see Figure 3.4). They crossed a-strain and b-strain mice to generate hybrid progeny that carried both strains of MHC-encoded protein throughout their bodies. The thymus of each hybrid mouse was then removed and the animal was irradiated to kill all its B and T cells. A new thymus from a b-strain mouse was transplanted into the hybrid mouse, and new bone-marrow stem cells were grafted into the mouse from another hybrid animal of the same kind.

In an ordinary hybrid mouse the hybrid stem cells would develop into mature T cells that respond collectively to antigen associated either with a-strain, MHC-encoded protein or with b-strain protein. In the experimental animals, however, only b-strain proteins were present on the nonlymphatic cells in the thymus, although both strains were still present throughout the rest of the body. Surprisingly, the investigators found that the mature T cells from such animals could respond to antigen only in association with b-strain, MHC-encoded protein, not to antigen in association with a-strain protein. Thus as the T cells developed in the b-strain thymus their receptors were apparently selected to recognize antigen only in association with the MHC-encoded proteins found in that organ. The T cells apparently

fail to recognize antigen associated with MHC-encoded protein that is foreign to the host's thymus.

Many hypotheses have been put forward to account for this unexpected finding, none of them yet completely satisfactory. Perhaps T-cell receptors must bind weakly to self-MHC-encoded proteins in the thymus before the T cells can mature and become functional. Subsequently the T cells whose receptors have the highest affinity for self-MHC-encoded proteins might undergo clonal abortion; the remaining T cells, with a low but still positive affinity for self-MHC-encoded proteins, would then be released into circulation. When antigen becomes bound to such a protein, however, the affinity of the receptor on the circulating T cells for the antigen might be substantially increased.

What about the strong response of T cells to foreign tissue graft? The favored explanation is that to the T cell a foreign-MHC-encoded protein looks much the same chemically as a complex of a self-MHC-encoded protein bound to an antigen. The explanation accounts for several observations. For example, the T-cell receptor that binds the self-MHC-encoded protein appears to be the same receptor that also binds the foreign protein. Furthermore, the receptor seems to have a predisposition for binding to antigen in the presence of either the

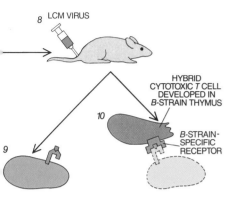

Figure 3.4 HYBRID MOUSE PROGENY were immunized against LCM virus (*1*), and cytotoxic *T* cells were isolated from the mice (*2*). The *T* cells were to kill cells infected with the virus from both *a*-strain and *b*-strain mice (*3*). The thymus was removed from another hybrid mouse, and all preexisting *T* cells and other lymphoid cells were killed by irradiating the animal (*4*). New bone-marrow stem cells were then obtained from another hybrid mouse (*5*), and the irradiated thymus of a *b*-strain mouse was transplanted into the thymectomized hybrid (*6*). The hybrid stem cells were then allowed to develop in the hybrid mouse with the *b*-strain thymus (*7*). When the experimentally constructed hybrid mouse was immunized against LCH virus (*8*), the *T* cells isolated were not able to kill virus-infected cells from *a*-strain mice (*9*), although they were able to kill such infected cells from *b*-strain mice (*10*).

class I protein or the class II protein, but not both, whether or not the MHC-encoded protein is foreign.

There has been much work seeking some basis for these receptor predispositions. So far, however, no one has observed any obvious differences between *T* cells restricted to one or the other class of MHC-encoded proteins. In 1984 Tonegawa and his colleagues did find a third kind of gene, called the gamma gene, that is rearranged by *T* cells. The properties of the genetic sequence suggest the protein it encodes is not part of the *T*-cell receptor as the receptor is currently understood. Nevertheless, the protein is expressed only in cytotoxic *T* cells, and so perhaps it contributes in some unsuspected way to the MHC-specificity of the cell that bears it.

If there is a chemical similarity between foreign-MHC-encoded protein and a complex of self-MHC-encoded protein and antigen, one might expect the antigen in the complex to be quite small. A small piece of antigen would also fit more readily into the binding cleft of the *T*-cell receptor than a large piece. Recent work by a number of groups, including Emil Unanue and his colleagues, Ronald H. Schwartz and his colleagues at the National Institute of Allergy and Infectious Diseases and our own group, in collaboration with Howard M. Grey of the National Jewish Center for Immunology and Respi-

ratory Medicine, has shown that the bound antigen is indeed small.

For example, we found that *T* cells respond to live cells incubated with an antigen, but they do not respond to the same antigen when it is added to the cells after they have been fixed with a chemical. When only a small fragment of the antigen is added to the chemically fixed cells, the *T* cell responds once again. The work confirms that the antigen-presenting cells to which a *T* cell can bind have already processed, or digested, the antigen in some way.

We must raise one final point. The existence of the *B* cell makes it clear that a system can be developed in which a receptor recognizes and binds free, native antigen. The binding eventually leads to clonal expansion and differentiation of the *B* cell, which gives rise to antibodies that are quite effective in marking the antigen for destruction. Why then has the *T* cell evolved such an elaborate system for recognizing antigen only in association with the products of the MHC?

There is a teleological answer to the question: The *T* cell is intended to react solely to antigen on a cellular target, and not to free antigen. A cytotoxic *T* cell, for example, is designed to kill virus-infected cells and thereby inhibit the growth and spread of the virus. Such a cell cannot kill a free virus particle, and so the resources of the *T* cell could be squandered if there were no means of directing its attention to a virus growing inside a nucleated cell. The immune system has therefore designed the *T*-cell receptor in such a way that it can bind a viral antigen only when it can also bind a self-MHC-encoded class I protein, which is present on the surface of every nucleated cell in the body.

Even more craftily, the immune system has designed receptors on helper *T* cells that are destined to interact primarily with the *B* cell and with other cells of the immune system. These receptors bind antigen only when it is associated with self-MHC-encoded class II proteins, which are expressed only on the surfaces of the *B* cells and the other immune cells. The immune system has thus evolved in such a way that both classes of MHC-encoded proteins serve as signposts for the *T* cell. They guide the *T* cell to antigen in precisely the places where the action of the *T* cell can be effective.

How *T* Cells See Antigen

On their own, these key actors in the immune response are blind. Other cells must break down foreign material and enfold it in the body's own proteins before displaying it to the T cells.

· · ·

Howard M. Grey, Alessandro Sette and Søren Buus
November, 1989

The human body is constantly fighting an imperceptible war against invading microbes and malignant cells. The battle is led by the immune system, which can eliminate or neutralize virtually any invader while sparing the body's own tissues at the same time. The main defenders are the white blood cells called lymphocytes, and the counterattack has at least two prongs. The more familiar one consists of the *B* cells, which react to antigen — distinctive foreign material — by secreting antibodies that bind to the invader. Bolstering the activity of the *B* cells, and supplementing it with a second defensive response, are the *T* cells. These lymphocytes help *B* cells to proliferate and secrete antibodies, and they also kill virus-infected and malignant cells directly.

A precise event triggers the immune response: a receptor molecule on the surface of a *B* cell or a *T* cell encounters the antigen to which the cell is programmed to respond and binds to some small part of it, thereby recognizing it as foreign. Aided by other elements of the immune system, the cell then multiplies and fulfills its role as an antibody-secreting *B* cell, a cytotoxic (cell-killing) *T* cell or a helper *T* cell, which secretes substances that mobilize the other cells. *B* cells perform this feat of recognition

on their own, interacting with antigens on bacteria or parasites without any intermediary. Yet isolated *T* cells are blind. What more do they need in order to see a foreign substance?

It has become clear during the past several decades that *T* cells have exacting requirements for recognizing antigen. Another kind of cell must act as a so-called accessory cell, chemically processing the antigen and presenting it to the *T* cell in association with certain of the accessory cell's own surface proteins, known as MHC molecules. Immunologists and molecular biologists are still vigorously probing the intricacies of antigen processing, the nature of the MHC molecules and the role they play in presenting antigen to *T* cells. We have already learned much about this key prelude to the immune response, however. What we know promises to lead to new ways of controlling the immune response. It may aid, for example, in the development of synthetic vaccines and of specific therapies for autoimmune diseases such as multiple sclerosis.

One of the first indications that *B* and *T* cells see antigen in fundamentally different ways came from work done 30 years ago by P. G. H. Gell and Baruj Benacerraf, who were then at New York University. They found that antibodies (and the cells making them) that were specific for a foreign protein in its normal, intricately folded form often ignored it after it had been denatured—disordered or unfolded. Yet the "cell-mediated" immune response, which is the work of T cells, was virtually identical for proteins in their normal and denatured forms. B and T cells were not known at the time, but these experiments suggested in retrospect that B cells and the antibodies they secrete must recognize antigen mainly by its shape, whereas T cells respond mostly to its makeup—to the sequence of amino acids in the protein chain, which would be identical regardless of how the molecule was folded.

Subsequently, the evidence mounted that T cells respond to antigen only when an accessory cell "presents" it (see Figure 4.1). Macrophages, the immune system's scavenger cells, were the first accessory cells to be identified; later, dendritic cells (specialized cells found in the lymph nodes and spleen), B cells themselves and, for some kinds of T cell reactions, any nucleated cell in the body were added to the list. It turned out that the activity of accessory cells, or antigen-presenting cells (APC's), explains why T cells have no interest in antigen shape: the APC's break down the antigen before presenting it, obscuring its shape and leaving only its distinctive amino acid sequence.

Several studies showed that APC's do more than simply capture antigen and display it on their surface. A technique introduced in 1981 by Emil R. Unanue, then at Harvard University, yielded the most compelling results. He and his colleagues exposed APC's to antigen and then, after varying intervals, "fixed" the cells with formaldehyde, which interrupted their metabolism. The workers then tested the cells' ability to present antigen to T cells and trigger their proliferation. APC's fixed before or immediately after they were exposed to antigen could not present it to T cells. In contrast, APC's that were incubated with antigen for an hour or more and then fixed were perfectly capable of doing so. These results and others suggested that, after exposure to antigen, accessory cells required time and energy before they could present antigen to T cells, probably because they had to modify it somehow first.

Other experiments shed light on this process by showing that certain weak bases strongly inhibit the ability of APC's to present antigen. The compounds are probably active in the endosomes, acidic com- partments within the cell where ingested material is broken down by proteolytic, or protein-cleaving, enzymes. Presumably by neutralizing the endosomes, the bases inhibit a cell's ability to degrade proteins. Later work showed that specific inhibitors of proteolytic enzymes also interfere with antigen presentation.

The possibility that cleavage of antigen into short fragments, or peptides, prepares it for presentation to T cells gained crucial support from an experiment done by Richard P. Shimonkevitz, Philippa C. Marrack and John W. Kappler, all of the National Jewish Center for Immunology and Respiratory Medicine in Denver, and one of us (Grey). The group showed that single peptides derived from a protein antigen could substitute for the intact protein in triggering a T cell response. The peptides clearly needed no further processing to do so, since they could be presented by APC's that had previously been fixed. Recently Stephane O. Demotz in our laboratory at Cytel actually isolated a processed antigen and determined that it is indeed a short peptide. In one account of antigen processing, then, an APC engulfs antigen and delivers it to acidic compartments within the cell, where it is broken down into small peptides, as short as 10 to 20 amino acids, before being returned to the cell membrane for recognition.

That is only a partial account of antigen processing, however. The steps it describes occur in the specific classes of antigen-presenting cells—B cells, macrophages and dendritic cells—that are specialized for processing foreign material taken in from the surrounding medium. The processing and presentation of such "exogenous" antigens generally leads to the activation of a specific population of T cells: the helper cells that aid B cells in making antibody.

Not all the antigens recognized by T cells originate outside the presenting cells, however. A cell that has been infected by a virus or has become malignant may synthesize distinctive, virus- or tumor-specific proteins. Virtually all cells in the body can present such internally synthesized proteins, and they do so to T cells belonging to the second major population: the cytotoxic T cells. These lymphocytes respond to "endogenous" antigens by killing the cells that produce them.

Until recently many workers assumed that such endogenous antigens did not need to be processed, since the intact proteins are often expressed on the surface of the abnormal cells. It seemed plausible

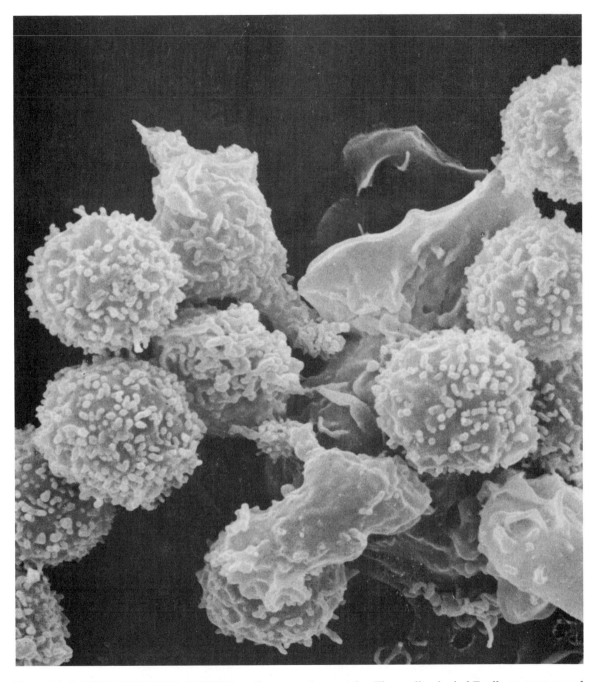

Figure 4.1 *T* CELLS RECOGNIZE ANTIGEN on the surface of a macrophage, a scavenger cell. The flat macrophage has ingested a bacterial protein, broken it down and displayed the pieces together with certain of the cell's surface proteins. The small, spherical *T* cells are programmed to recognize the bacterial antigens but can only do so with the macrophage's assistance. (Micrograph is by Morten H. Nielsen and Ole Werdelin.)

that cytotoxic *T* cells, unlike helper cells, might be able to respond directly to intact antigen. Yet Alain Townsend of the John Radcliffe Hospital in Oxford found in 1985 that cytotoxic cells capable of killing cells infected with a virus could also kill uninfected cells into which a mere fragment of a viral gene had been introduced. These genetically engineered cells produced only a small fraction of the corresponding viral protein found on the infected cells. The cytotoxic cells nonetheless responded identically to both molecules. Later Townsend induced a cytotoxic response with uninfected APC's that had merely been incubated with a short antigenic peptide, confirming that cytotoxic cells, like helper cells, recognize a fragment of antigen and not the complete protein.

Other experiments indicated, however, that infected cells process endogenous antigens by a mechanism quite different from the one that prepares antigen for recognition by helper cells. The weak bases that blocked processing for helper *T* cell recognition and pointed to a central role for endosomes in that processing pathway had no effect on antigen presentation to cytotoxic *T* cells. Moreover, when an antigenic protein was added to a culture containing APC's and antigen-specific cytotoxic *T* cells, nothing happened. The killer cells were able to recognize and respond to the protein, however, when it was microinjected into the cytoplasm — the fluid interior medium — of the presenting cells.

The data are not yet completely definitive, but they are most compatible with a picture in which endogenous antigen is processed in the cytoplasm rather than within endosomes. Once the protein has been degraded in the cytoplasm, the fragments are somehow moved into the interior of a vesicle, a sac that shuttles between the cell interior and its surface. The peptides are then transported to the cell surface for recognition by killer *T* cells.

This second processing pathway, specialized for antigens made by the APC itself, could be the immune system's way of ensuring that a foreign organism cannot elude it by adopting a Trojan-horse strategy. Even if the pathogen is hidden within a cell, the body will process the novel proteins and make them visible to the *T* cells.

In addition, the existence of two separate pathways of antigen processing, one for exogenous antigens and one for endogenous antigens, makes biological sense: each pathway leads to the appropriate *T* cell response (see Figure 4.2). A bacterial protein taken up by a *B* cell from its surroundings and processed by the exogenous pathway elicits *T* cell

help, which enables the *B* cell to produce antibodies for combating the infection. A foreign or abnormal protein made by a renegade cell, in contrast, leads to the killing of the errant cell by cytotoxic *T* cells.

Once it has been processed, antigen is displayed on the surface of the accessory cell together with proteins of the cell's own making. They are known as MHC proteins, after the major histocompatibility gene complex, a cluster of more than a dozen genes. The cluster is a hot spot of genetic variability, so that the MHC proteins encoded by a given set of genes almost always differ from one individual to the next. The molecules do fall into two broad classes, however, according to their structure and their role in *T* cell stimulation. Class II MHC proteins, found mainly on the surface of *B* cells, macrophages and dendritic cells, figure in the presentation of antigen to helper *T* cells. Class I proteins, found on almost all nucleated cells in the body, play the same role for cytotoxic *T* cells.

The current picture of MHC molecules and their part in stimulating the *T* cell response is the product of more than three decades of investigation, beginning in the mid-1950's with studies of tissue grafts. Investigators found that when tissue from one animal was transferred to another one with different MHC proteins, the immune system of the recipient rejected the graft in an extraordinarily intense reaction, one that was later traced to *T* cells. It appeared that the immune system, and its *T* cell arm in particular, is "tuned" to recognizing MHC molecules. Clearly, though, their normal immunologic function had to be something other than graft rejection. After all, grafts are rare in nature.

An early hint of a normal function for MHC proteins came from experiments done in the 1960's by Hugh O. McDevitt, who was then at the National Institute for Medical Research in England, and Benacerraf. They showed that the genes of the MHC affected an animal's ability to mount an immune response to certain simple antigens. An animal carrying one variant of a particular MHC gene might respond vigorously to a given antigen; another animal carrying a different variant might not respond at all. In these responder and nonresponder strains, the MHC seemed to function as "immune response" genes.

How might these genes affect the immune response? The most obvious explanation was that they encoded the *T* cells' own receptor molecules. In 1973, however, Alan S. Rosenthal and Ethan M.

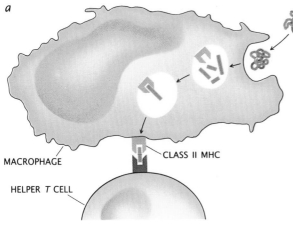

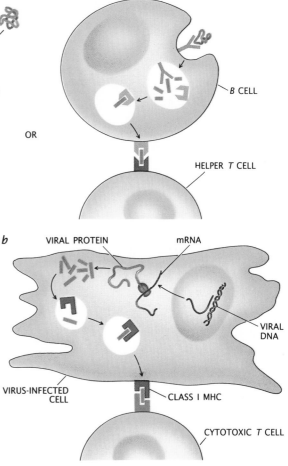

Figure 4.2 ANTIGEN IS PROCESSED by one of two pathways, depending on its origin. Foreign material from outside the cell is engulfed by a specialized cell (*a*), often a macrophage (*left*) or a *B* cell (*right*). The cell breaks down the material in an intracellular compartment and links the processed antigen to class II MHC molecules. The complexes are transported to the cell surface and displayed there to helper *T* cells. Abnormal proteins made within a virus-infected or malignant cell (*b*) are broken down in the cell's internal medium. Only then do the fragments move into a vesicle, or sac, where they join class I MHC molecules and are carried to the cell surface for display to cytotoxic *T* cells.

Shevach of the National Institute of Allergy and Infectious Diseases made an observation that linked the MHC to the function of the accessory cells. They mated a guinea-pig strain that responded well to one antigen and poorly to a second antigen with a strain that showed the reciprocal pattern, responding poorly to the first antigen and well to the second. The offspring—having inherited a gene for responsiveness from each parent—could mount a strong response to both antigens. But when the workers extracted *T* cells from the hybrid animals and mixed them with APC's and antigen in culture, the helper *T* cell response depended on the origin of the accessory cells.

In the presence of APC's that had also come from the hybrid animals, the *T* cells responded to both antigens, as expected. When the APC's had been isolated from the parental strains, however, the *T* cells reacted only to the antigen to which the parental strain had also responded. The cells seemed blind to the other antigen. It appeared that the MHC genes exerted their effect not through the *T* cells themselves (under the right conditions the *T* cells of the hybrid animals were perfectly capable of responding to both antigens) but through the APC's. Somehow accessory cells carrying the nonresponder genes were unable to present one of the antigens—a phenomenon for which the mechanism has only recently been elucidated.

Meanwhile studies of cytotoxic *T* cells led to the conclusion that *T* cells recognize not only foreign antigen but also the MHC-encoded proteins on the accessory cells. In 1974, for example, Rolf M. Zinkernagel and Peter C. Doherty of the Australian National University exposed T cells that had responded to antigen presented by cells carrying a particular variant of class I MHC protein to the same antigen presented by cells bearing a different MHC variant. First, the workers infected a mouse with a virus, stimulating cytotoxic T cells targeted to the virus-infected cells. Then they extracted the specific T cells and exposed them in vitro to virus-infected cells from other mice.

Zinkernagel and Doherty found that if the class I MHC proteins on the surface of these new infected cells differed from those of the original mouse, the cells escaped T cell killing. The workers interpreted the results as showing that an animal's T cells had to recognize two entities in order to respond: both an antigen and a specific MHC protein — one that is characteristic of the animal's own cells. Confirmed by many other experiments, this requirement for co-recognition of antigen and a "self" MHC molecule became known as MHC restriction.

This MHC restriction of the T cell response presented a new puzzle. B cells, after all, are activated by the fit of a single key (the antigen) into a single lock (the receptor on the B cell surface). What might be the molecular design of the T cell's double-key system? One theory held that T cells bear two independent receptor molecules, one specific for antigen and the other for a self-MHC protein. A second theory postulated that T cells carry a single receptor molecule capable of identifying both antigen and MHC. Proponents of each theory raised indirect evidence in its favor; the controversy was settled in favor of the one-receptor model when a single T cell receptor was shown to be specific for both antigen and self-MHC (see Chapter 3, "The T Cell and Its Receptor," by Philippa Marrack and John Kappler).

The existence of a single receptor suggested that the processed antigen and the MHC molecule might form a complex — a single entity that would fit a single recognition site in the T cell receptor. In effect, the MHC protein would act as the primary receptor for processed antigen; the resulting complex would then interact with a second receptor, on the T cell. Because both the antigen and the MHC would contribute to shaping the molecular characteristics of the complex, the proposed mechanism would elegantly explain T cells' specificity for both MHC and antigen. It might also explain the puzzle

early studies had posed: How do certain MHC genes render an individual blind to specific antigens? In this new picture, those genes might encode proteins unable to bind and present particular peptides.

Ronald H. Schwartz of the National Institute of Allergy and Infectious Diseases provided compelling but indirect evidence in favor of complex formation. He studied the ability of mice belonging to different MHC strains to react to variants of a particular protein. He found that whereas a specific variant might elicit a T cell response in one strain but not in a second one, a difference of a few amino acids in the protein's sequence might make it visible to the immune system of the second strain. Schwartz argued that such results were best explained by supposing that the protein — or a peptide cleaved from it — had to bind to MHC molecules before it could trigger a response. The slight difference in amino acid sequence was what was needed for the peptide to bind to the MHC molecules of the second strain.

In 1985 Unanue and his colleagues at Washington University were the first to demonstrate complex formation directly, by means of a technique called equilibrium dialysis. A chamber containing an antigenic peptide was separated by a semipermeable membrane from another chamber containing the class II MHC molecule that restricted the immune response to the antigen. The antigen — by far the smaller molecule — could pass through the membrane, but the MHC protein was confined on one side. All else being equal, the antigen should have diffused through the membrane until its concentration in both chambers was the same. Instead its concentration grew larger on the side that also contained the MHC protein. Evidently, the molecules were binding to each other.

Our group demonstrated the same kind of interaction for a variety of peptides and class II MHC molecules. We also showed that the binding is critical for an immune response: T cells recognize complexes of MHC and antigen. Adopting a technique developed in Harden M. McConnell's laboratory at Stanford University, we embedded antigen-MHC complexes into an artificial lipid membrane — a simulated cell membrane. For comparison, we also prepared membrane containing uncomplexed MHC, bathed in free antigen. The preformed complexes stimulated antigen-specific T cells some 20,000 times more efficiently than did the uncomplexed MHC and antigen.

For such complexes to have a role in the normal immune response, they must be quite stable: in any individual only a few *T* cells bear receptors specific for a given antigen, so that after an individual's exposure to the antigen it may take some time before a specific *T* cell encounters an APC bearing the antigen-MHC complex. The success of our experiment suggested that the complexes are indeed stable, since it took us more than a day to isolate antigen-MHC complexes and embed them in the lipid membrane. Direct measurements of the complexes' dissociation rates confirmed their stability: at body temperature their half-life was about 10 hours.

Compelling as the evidence of complex formation was, not everyone accepted the further proposal that a failure of some MHC proteins to bind certain antigens underlies the genetic unresponsiveness investigators such as Rosenthal and Shevach had studied. Experiments with different antigens did not always support Rosenthal and Shevach's conclusion that such immunologic blind spots reflect a deficit in the antigen-presenting cells. Also, some workers pointed out that it was hard to see how a single MHC protein could act as a specific receptor for myriad structurally distinct antigenic peptides.

After all, each individual has at most about a dozen MHC proteins. How could the MHC proteins be selective when each one must bind a sizable part of a vast universe of potential antigens? In this view, antigen-MHC complexes, if they existed, had to form nonspecifically. Variations in immune responsiveness had to reflect something other than selective binding.

Some investigators proposed instead that the MHC influences the immune response by shaping the repertoire of functional *T* cells. *T* cells mature in the thymus gland, and in the process they interact with the MHC proteins on the surface of accessory cells in the thymus. During this thymic "education," the *T* cells learn to recognize antigen only in association with the body's own MHC molecules. At the same time, it is thought, *T* cells that bind too avidly to self-MHC—and hence pose the threat of an autoimmune reaction—are eliminated or at least inactivated. Conceivably, a particular variant of a self-MHC protein might lead to the elimination of all the *T* cells capable of reacting to a particular antigen. Any individual inheriting the corresponding MHC

gene would display the same hole in the *T* cell repertoire.

We tested the relative influences on immune responsiveness of MHC binding and holes in the *T* cell repertoire by comparing peptides' ability to bind to a mouse MHC molecule with their ability to induce an immune response (see Figure 4.3). Of a set of 14 peptides—which in sum represented an entire protein molecule—five could bind to the MHC protein; three of those five, we found, could then trigger a *T* cell response in animals of the same MHC strain. None of the peptides that failed to bind could stimulate a response.

The selectivity of the MHC proteins, then, does shape the immune response. But not every peptide that can bind to a self-MHC elicits a response; some antigens that bind fail to stimulate a response, apparently because *T* cells able to recognize the antigen-MHC complex are absent. Both theories of how the MHC genes influence the immune response appear to be correct. The selectivity of MHC proteins in binding antigens combines with holes in the *T* cell arsenal to set the boundaries of an individual's immune responsiveness.

The earlier objection to the notion of MHC proteins as specific antigen receptors remained unanswered, however: How could an MHC protein selectively bind many—but not all—antigens? We found that a typical MHC molecule can indeed bind between 10 and 20 percent of the peptide fragments from any given protein molecule. We also identified a possible basis for this broad but selective binding: peptides bound by a particular MHC molecule turned out to share certain simple structural features (see Figure 4.4).

One MHC molecule, for example, bound peptides that all shared a motif of repeated hydrophobic residues—amino acids with an affinity for a nonwater medium. Another MHC molecule bound peptides that had in common a trio of positively charged residues. Perhaps such diverse, broad specificities give an individual's array of MHC proteins the ability to bind and present the widest possible variety of antigens, so that a foreign substance is unlikely to slip through the immune system's defenses.

Vivid confirmation that MHC molecules serve as receptors for processed antigen exported to the cell surface came in 1987, when Don C. Wiley and his colleagues at Harvard University solved the three-dimensional structure of a class I MHC mole-

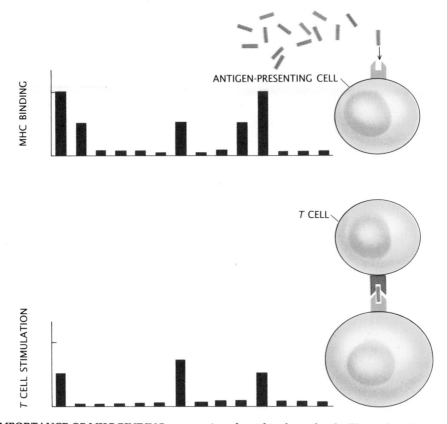

Figure 4.3 IMPORTANCE OF MHC BINDING to an antigen's ability to stimulate a *T* cell response was assessed by the authors. They synthesized 14 peptides representing fragments of a protein and measured the affinity of each one for a mouse MHC molecule (*top*). Five of the peptides bound to the molecule. Three of the five could stimulate a *T* cell response in a mouse of the same strain (*bottom*). Binding to an MHC protein appears to be necessary, but not sufficient, for a peptide to trigger an immune response.

cule. The most striking feature of the structure, determined from the diffraction pattern of X rays trained on a crystal of the protein, was a cleft on the top of the molecule, where it would face outward from the cell surface (see Figure 4.5). Two helical regions of the protein form the walls of the cleft; so-called beta sheets, in which the protein chain folds back and forth in a plane, form the cleft's floor.

The cleft *looks* like the binding site for an antigenic peptide. What is more, many of the variable amino acids that distinguish a particular MHC protein in different individuals and affect immune responsiveness turn out to be clustered on the inside walls and floor of the cleft. Such amino acids presumably influence the protein's peptide-binding ability; one would therefore expect them to mark the binding site.

A second observation also pointed to the cleft as the peptide-binding site and raised an intriguing new possibility about the function of MHC molecules. The cleft was not empty: in it Wiley and his colleagues identified another molecular entity. The material must have been bound to the MHC molecules when they were crystallized; presumably, it was a piece of processed antigen.

Paul M. Allen of Washington University and our own group have confirmed that the binding site on MHC proteins of accessory cells is routinely occupied. Acid treatment of class II MHC molecules purified from *B* cells released peptides that later could rebind specifically to the MHC molecules. What is

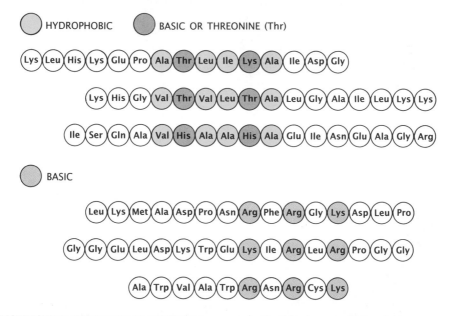

Figure 4.4 DISTINCTIVE STRUCTURAL MOTIFS characterize peptides able to bind to particular MHC proteins. The upper three peptides all bind well to one MHC molecule; the lower three all bind well to another such molecule. Peptides in each cluster share a common pattern defined by the chemical properties of their constituent amino acids.

more, Townsend and his co-workers recently showed that a cell cannot even assemble class I MHC molecules properly unless a peptide is present during the final stages of the protein's folding process. It seems likely that these omnipresent peptides are fragments of the body's own proteins, produced within the cell or captured from its surroundings, that have been processed and presented by the same mechanisms that display foreign antigens.

That proposal is consistent with the theory of immune surveillance, which holds that killer *T* cells constantly monitor the other cells of the body for the appearance of tumor or viral antigens and promptly eliminate any cell expressing them. By continuously processing and presenting their own antigens, cells in effect invite inspection by the immune system, so that it can quickly detect any aberration.

This scenario of constant self-scrutiny suggests an answer to the inevitable question about antigen presentation to *T* cells: Why does it need to be so elaborate? Why do *T* cells not recognize antigen directly, as *B* cells do, instead of requiring it to be broken down and displayed in the context of MHC molecules? For cytotoxic *T* cells, one answer is that MHC restriction targets them to the body's own tissue, where—being killer cells—they are designed to act. Because the cells are "interested" in self-MHC as well as antigen, they look for antigen in precisely the setting in which they can respond effectively to it.

For the equally complex scheme of antigen presentation to helper *T* cells, one might invoke an evolutionary explanation. Cell-mediated immunity appears to be ancient; even organisms as primitive as sponges can recognize and prevent invasion by cells from different species. Thus, *T* cells may have originated as killer cells, but even when they acquired an additional, helper role, they retained a disposition to look for antigen on the cell surface, in association with the body's own proteins. Over the course of evolution, this interest in self-proteins became adapted to the helper cells' function, so that class II MHC proteins now guide these *T* cells to a site where they can be most effective—to *B* cells, the primary target of *T* cell help.

Even though the picture of antigen processing and presentation is far from complete, understanding of the phenomenon has advanced dramat-

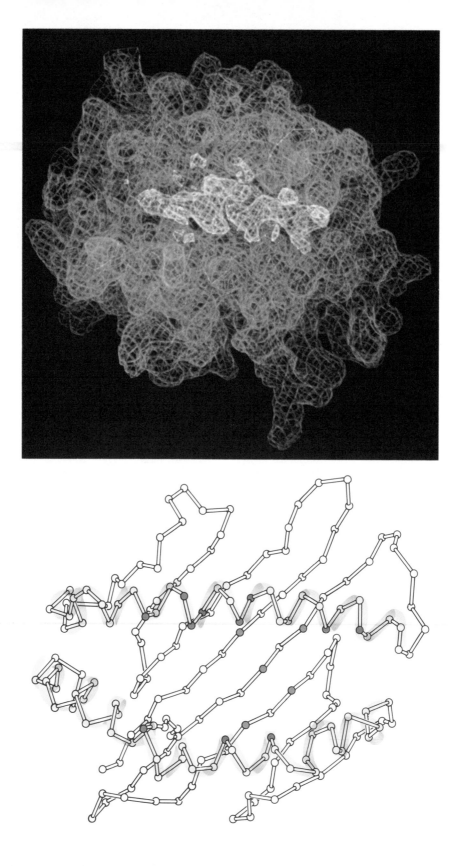

ically. The result is likely to be an improved ability to manipulate the immune system for clinical purposes: to stimulate immunity with vaccines and selectively suppress it in autoimmune diseases.

Traditionally, vaccines have consisted of the whole pathogenic organism, live or killed, or a protein extracted from it. For some diseases, such as malaria, that approach is not feasible, and some whole-organism vaccines have risky side effects. In such cases vaccine developers are now trying to design synthetic peptides (representing only a small part of the actual antigen) that will trigger an equivalent immune response. To do so, the peptides must stimulate helper and cytotoxic *T* cells as well as *B* cells, and so it is critical that these antigens bind to MHC molecules in spite of individual variation. The deepening understanding of MHC-antigen interactions will surely help guide the design of such peptide vaccines.

It may also help in treating insulin-dependent diabetes, rheumatoid arthritis and multiple sclerosis —diseases in which the immune system loses its ability to discriminate self from nonself and responds to the body's own molecules. Some of these diseases almost exclusively affect people carrying specific MHC genes. The corresponding MHC proteins may play a role in the diseases by presenting self-antigens in a way that induces an immune response.

MHC-based technology should make it possible to develop compounds that bind very strongly to the disease-associated MHC proteins. By blocking the binding of self-antigens, such compounds might suppress the autoimmune response. It is already possible to arrest some of these diseases by means of an immunosuppressive agent (such as cyclosporine), which blocks the immune response generally. A blocker targeted to a specific MHC variant, however, would have the advantage of leaving the immune system largely intact and able to defend the body against external threats. Growing understanding of antigen processing and presentation may thus give the fight against autoimmune diseases some of the immune system's own precision and power.

Figure 4.5 ANTIGEN-BINDING CLEFT of a class I MHC molecule is shown in two images based on X-ray analysis of the protein: a computer model (*top*) and a diagram (*bottom*), where the cleft lies between the two helixes. The discovery of a separate substance (*orange in the computer image*) lodged in the cleft supported the proposal that it is the binding site for antigen. In addition, many of the variable amino acids (*red in the diagram*) that affect a particular MHC molecule's antigen-binding capability are clustered in the cleft. Don C. Wiley and Pamela J. Bjorkman, Mark A. Saper, Boudjema Samraoui, William S. Bennett and Jack L. Strominger determined the molecular structure.

REGULATORY AND EFFECTOR MECHANISMS OF THE IMMUNE RESPONSE

. . .

Introduction

Understanding the specificity mechanisms of the immune system has been the major goal of a century of immunological research. Although much work remains to be done in this area, there is no doubt that remarkable progress has been made in the field. However, recognition of foreign antigens is valuable only if that recognition can be linked to mechanisms through which the recognized entity can be destroyed, eliminated or neutralized. Furthermore, the vast number of cells that can participate in an immune response and the processes of cell proliferation and differentiation that are key to a successful response require sophisticated regulatory mechanisms through which cells can communicate with one another. The linked fields of immunologic regulation and effector mechanisms have been the subject of strikingly increased attention and promise to become the dominant aspects of immunological research in the future.

Among the most recent important advances in immunology have been the purification, molecular cloning and functional characterization of a wide array of regulatory proteins produced by T cells and other cells of the immune system. These molecules are variously known as lymphokines or cytokines. One of the proteins that regulate the growth of T cells and B cells is interleukin-2 (IL-2), the subject of Chapter 5, by Kendall A. Smith. Others are IL-3, IL-4, IL-5, IL-6, granulocyte-macrophage colony stimulating factor, (GM-CSF), and interferon gamma. An immune system-derived protein that can inhibit the growth of a variety of cell types, including tumor cells, is the subject of Chapter 6, "Tumor Necrosis Factor," by Lloyd J. Old.

These proteins have been purified and the genes encoding them have been cloned and expressed. Further, it has been shown that these molecules act on their target cells by binding to high-affinity receptors expressed on those cells. The structure of the receptors and the means through which growth factor–receptor interactions lead to biologic functions are now issues of central importance in the study of immune responses.

The use of the pure proteins and of antibodies to them as tools to study the function of lymphokines and related regulatory and effector molecules in the immune system has yielded much exciting information. Among the major organizing principles that have emerged is that the relatively straightforward classification of lymphokines by function is a vast oversimplification. Individual lymphokines have a multiplicity of functions and the same function is often exerted by more than one lymphokine. Among the major challenges that must now be faced is to understand how these proteins actually function physiologically, how their production is controlled and what contribution they make to both normal responses and to the abnormal responses that are observed in various diseases.

Equally exciting is the potential that these agents have in therapy. Several of them have been considered for use in patients with a variety of disorders, such as in depressed bone-marrow function due to disease or to chemotherapy for cancer and in the treatment of individuals with a variety of malignancies. Finally, the possibility of neutralizing the function of some of these molecules to treat a variety of inflammatory and allergic conditions is being given serious consideration.

The immune system has a variety of effector mechanisms through which it may eliminate or neutralize microbes and other potentially pathogenic agents. Among these are the complement system, a complex series of interacting enzymes that is called into play by the binding of antibody to antigen and which has many biologic effects, including the physical destruction of bacteria and of cells that bear foreign antigens. Another of the most striking and effective means that the immune system can utilize is the capacity of a specialized set of T lymphocytes to recognize and kill cells that express certain antigen-derived peptides bound to class I MHC molecules. The mechanisms of such killing are discussed in Chapter 7, "How Killer Cells Kill," by John Ding-E Young and Zanvil A. Cohn.

Killer cells are of particular importance in immune responses against virus-infected cells. The recent recognition that many tumors of humans have accumulated mutations in a series of genes suggests that killer cells may have targets for recognition of such cells. Indeed, evidence that tumor cells have often extinguished the expression of class I MHC molecules suggests that "successful" tumors are ones that have escaped the attention of killer cells by disabling the mechanism through which antigen-derived peptides are displayed on the cell surface.

Ding-E Young and Cohn discuss the mechanisms that killer cells use to destroy their targets. They pay particular attention to perforin, a T cell–derived protein that can be inserted into the membranes of target cells and leads to the formation of pores within such cells. These pores result in the death of the target cells through osmotic lysis. There is reason to believe that perforin insertion into target cells is but one of several mechanisms through which killer T cells can destroy target cells bearing antigens for which their receptors are specific.

Chapters 5, 6 and 7 provide an introduction to the complex and important area of immunology that deals with the regulatory interactions among immunocompetent cells and with the means through which these cells protect the host against the consequences of infection and other types of pathogenic attack.

Interleukin-2

The first hormone of the immune system to be recognized, it helps the body to mount a defense against microorganisms by triggering the multiplication of only those cells that attack an invader.

• • •

Kendall A. Smith
March, 1990

Ever since Edward Jenner introduced vaccination in 1797 as a means of preventing smallpox, biologists have been fascinated and mystified by the immune system. During the past two centuries, investigators have slowly learned that the activity of the immune system depends on a symphony of highly specialized types of cells in the blood and tissues, each cell type performing a unique function. Yet as the roster of immune cells grew, it remained unclear how this unconnected multitude of cells was able to orchestrate its activities into a selective defense against diseases. Consequently, until recently, immunity was a mysterious phenomenon, and immunology seemed hopelessly complex and esoteric even to biologists in other disciplines.

Within the past 10 years, however, immunology has been transformed by the demonstration that the immune system is regulated by hormones in much the same way as are most other organ systems. Today immunology is no longer a science set apart by a specialized vocabulary and array of mechanisms. Instead the discovery and characterization of the interleukins, the hormones of the immune system, have made it clear that the immune response operates according to the same principles governing the classic hormones and their receptors.

Interleukin-2 (IL-2) was the first of the new immunologic hormones to be discovered and characterized. Although eight interleukins are now recognized by immunologists, the functions of some of these are undetermined or are not connected directly to immunity; IL-2, in contrast, is pivotal for the generation of an effective immune response. Accordingly, an understanding of IL-2 and its receptors opens the way for the development of therapeutic approaches to a wide range of conditions, including cancer, autoimmune disorders, chronic infectious diseases, acquired immunodeficiency syndrome (AIDS) and organ-transplant rejection.

An understanding of the role of IL-2 has done much to explain the specific properties of the immune system. Just as the nervous system senses and responds to changes in light, sound and other environmental stimuli, so the immune system senses and responds to the invasion of molecules in the form of foreign microorganisms, such as bacteria, viruses, fungi and parasites. To accomplish its tasks, the immune system combines three novel characteristics. First, immune reactivity is both highly specific and extremely diverse, properties that enable the body to recognize and respond to any possible microbe or foreign molecule (antigen). The immune system also has an exquisite ability to discriminate between the self and the nonself and only rarely turns on the body's own normal tissues. Finally, the immune system has a memory: after the initial exposure to an antigen, mysterious changes in the immune system make it capable of responding much more quickly and forcefully to reexposures.

Niels K. Jerne, who received the Nobel Prize for medicine in 1984, laid the groundwork for the current understanding of the immune system in 1955 while working at the California Institute of Technology. He proposed that immune reactivity is based on the Darwinian principle of natural selection. It was already known that antibody molecules in the blood reacted specifically with antigens; Jerne suggested that everyone carries an initially small number of antibodies against every possible antigen. When an antigen enters the body, the antibodies capable of binding to it are positively selected (to use Darwin's terminology) and increase in number.

Four years later another Nobel laureate, Sir Macfarlane Burnet of the Walter and Eliza Hall Institute of Medical Research in Melbourne, gave Jerne's natural-selection theory a cellular basis in a small book entitled *The Clonal Selection Theory of Acquired Immunity*. In it, Burnet proposed that each antibody molecule is the product of a single cell. According to Burnet, the antigen reacts directly with the antibody-producing cell to stimulate antibody production. (This idea was first suggested in 1905 by Paul Ehrlich, the pioneering immunologist and Nobelist.) Implicit in Burnet's hypothesis was the idea that after selective activation by an antigen, the antibody-producing cell proliferated to form a clone, a set of cells with one common ancestor.

At the time of Burnet's proposal, the cells responsible for reacting with antigens were unknown, although it was fairly certain that the white blood cells called plasma cells produced large amounts of antibodies. Lymphocytes, the predominant cells in the lymph nodes, were the most obvious candidates to react initially with antigens and thereby serve as the precursors for plasma cells, but lymphocytes were generally believed to be incapable of proliferating. Yet only one year later, in 1960, Peter C. Nowell of the University of Pennsylvania discovered that lymphocytes could proliferate, given the proper chemical stimulus.

In the decade after Burnet's hypothesis and Nowell's discovery, a sound cellular understanding of the immune system was established. Lymphocytes were found to be of two major types, B cells and T cells. B cells, which are derived from bone marrow, express antibody molecules on their surface, as Burnet had envisioned. Experiments by Gustav Nossal of the Hall Institute and by Jerne and Albert A. Nordin of the University of Pittsburgh demonstrated that when stimulated by a specific antigen, each B cell becomes a plasma cell that secretes antibodies with a single specificity.

T cells, which mature in the thymus, do not produce antibodies, but they do bear specific antigen receptors on their surface that strikingly resemble antibody molecules and that selectively bind antigen. Like B cells, T cells react to antigen stimulation by secreting molecules that mediate their immune function. On the basis of the molecules they secrete, T cells have been subcategorized as helper T cells and cytotoxic T cells. Today it is clear that helper T cells fulfill their role by secreting interleukins. Cytotoxic T cells, in contrast, make direct contact with infected cells and, by secreting toxic molecules, kill the cells and the microbes they contain.

T cells, in particular, turned out to serve as a good laboratory model of the immune response. When an antigen is injected into the body, the only detectable immune reaction is against that antigen specifically. In culture, T cell proliferation is also antigen-specific: only those cells that react with a given antigen survive and multiply. For this reason, the short-term culture of T cells was adopted in 1965 as a test-tube reproduction of the immune response. Also, the behavior of the cultured T cells helped to explain the phenomenon of immune memory: exposure to an antigen selectively increases the number of cells capable of responding to it in the future.

Immunologists had always assumed that antigen was the sole stimulus for B and T cell division. This assumption, which became dogma, had to be overturned before immunology could proceed to a more detailed and accurate description of how the immune system works.

The beginnings of the current understanding of the mechanisms responsible for stimulating lymphocyte growth can be traced back to 1965, when two teams of investigators at the Royal Victoria Hospital in Montreal, Shinpei Kasakura and Louis Lowenstein and, independently, J. Gordon and Lloyd D. MacLean, published papers simultaneously in *Nature*. Both teams reported that culture media "conditioned" by proliferating lymphocytes contained an unidentified substance that enhanced lymphocyte growth when antigen was present.

Many reports about these mysterious growth-enhancing substances appeared during the next decade. Nevertheless, most immunologists ignored these reports and continued to maintain that antigens were the sole agents responsible for lymphocyte proliferation. At most, the factor in the lymphocyte-conditioned medium was thought simply to amplify proliferation that had already been triggered by an antigen. With this idea in mind, various investigators had published several papers by the early 1970's that described ways of growing lymphocytes in culture for prolonged periods through the repetitive addition of antigen. It was possible to stimulate the proliferation of cultured lymphocytes for as long as four months by these techniques, and the lymphocytes retained their antigen specificity.

Immunologists doubted that a factor released by cells could specifically stimulate lymphocyte division because such a factor, it seemed, should amplify the proliferation of all lymphocytes regardless of whether they had encountered their specific antigen. In 1976, however, Doris A. Morgan, working with Francis W. Ruscetti in Robert C. Gallo's laboratory at the National Cancer Institute (NCI) in Bethesda, Md., reported that normal human T cells could be cultured without antigen for up to nine months, provided that a lymphocyte-conditioned medium was added to the cultures at regular intervals.

Actually, Morgan's observation was serendipitous. A self-proclaimed novice in lymphocyte culture methods, Morgan was trained in hematology and in hematopoiesis (the process by which blood cells develop). While trying to establish long-term cultures of leukemia cells, Morgan employed a lymphocyte-conditioned medium as a stimulant because lymphocytes were known to release factors that promoted the growth of the early blood-forming cells. Much to her initial anguish, the cells from leukemia patients that grew in the lymphocyte-conditioned medium appeared to be normal T cells instead of leukemia cells. For immunologists, however, her findings were important in that they suggested that some kind of factor in the conditioned medium other than antigen was responsible for T cell growth.

Although Morgan's report appeared in the prominent journal *Science*, its significance was lost on most of the immunology community. Morgan and her co-workers were well known in hematology and virology circles but were unfamiliar to most immunologists. The title of the paper stressed that the cultivated T cells had come from bone marrow, which meant that they might be immature or otherwise unrepresentative of most T cells. More important, the cultured cells were not shown to perform any antigen-specific functions, and immunologists were traditionally indifferent to phenomena that lacked antigen specificity.

Like Morgan, I was trained in hematology and hematopoiesis rather than in immunology. As a postdoctoral fellow, I had worked with George Mathe of the Institute of Cancer and Genetic Research in Villejuif, France, who was one of the first investigators to try to treat leukemia with immunotherapy. I had become intrigued by the possibility of stimulating the growth of cytotoxic lymphocytes to kill leukemia cells. In 1974, therefore, as assistant professor of medicine at Dartmouth Medical School, I initiated a research program directed toward understanding the fundamental determinants of cellular proliferation. By 1976 my colleagues and I had demonstrated that cytotoxic T cells could kill mouse leukemia cells in culture, and yet we were frustrated by our inability to maintain T cells in culture for more than a few days. We therefore decided to try new methods to achieve long-term, antigen-specific T cell growth.

Unencumbered by immunology's dogmas, we combined the methods that others had already tested. First we vaccinated mice repeatedly with irradiated tumor cells to expand the population of tumor-reactive T cells in the animals. T cells from the mice were then mixed with tumor cells in tissue culture; in this short-term culture, only those T cells reacting with tumor antigen would survive and proliferate. After one to two weeks the surviving T cells were transferred to a lymphocyte-conditioned medium similar to that described by Morgan. Steven Gillis, who was a first-year graduate student at the time, was the first in the laboratory to succeed at creating long-term cultures of T cells.

In short, despite the prevailing opinion that this approach would fail because we had removed the specific tumor antigen, we saw the long-term growth of tumor-antigen-specific cytotoxic T lymphocytes in the conditioned medium. Our paper appeared in *Nature* in July, 1977. In contrast to the lack of attention accorded Morgan's paper, the immunologic community was very interested in our report because it emphasized the culture of functional, antigen-specific T cells.

Our success suggested that we might be able to validate Burnet's clonal hypothesis directly by developing clones of antigen-specific cells, all derived from a single cell. Again, the prevailing opinion predicted that this would be an almost impossible task because single cells usually grow poorly (if at all) in culture. Yet the addition of the lymphocyte-conditioned medium led to T cell clones with surprising efficiency. Each clone showed antigen-specific cytotoxicity that could be ascribed to the clone's descent from a single cell. We reported the derivation of the first monoclonal cytotoxic T cell lines in 1979, 20 years after Burnet had formulated his clonal-selection theory.

Fundamental problems in immunology that had been impossible to approach with heterogeneous populations of lymphocytes were solved with antigen-specific cloned cell lines. For example, the ability to grow unlimited numbers of identical T cells led to a molecular characterization of the T cell antigen receptor. It was also instrumental in demonstrating unequivocally that a protein structure called the major histocompatibility complex plays an essential role in the recognition of antigen by T cells. The ability to grow clones of helper and cytotoxic T cells was important for identifying the molecular mechanisms underlying the cells' activities. In brief, the ability to derive and manipulate T cell clones in culture provided detailed molecular proof of Burnet's clonal-selection hypothesis.

Our first experiments provided the initial insight into how the selection of a clone by an antigen-specific process can initiate cell proliferation that depends only on a growth factor. The most logical explanation is that when a lymphocyte is activated by antigen, it develops a unique capacity to respond to the growth factor; the vast majority of lymphocytes (which do not respond to the same antigen) remain inactive.

My colleagues and I conducted a series of experiments to test this theory, and we proudly submitted the results to one of the most prestigious immunology journals in 1978. To our chagrin, however, the notion of a growth factor was still too heretical: everyone "knew" that antigen was the only thing that stimulated T cells to proliferate. The reviewers, it seemed, were skeptical and insisted on detailed biochemical information about the factor that we did not then have.

Consequently, we devoted our efforts to defining both the biological and biochemical characteristics of the T cell growth factor. Although lymphocyte growth factors had been described since 1965, no one had developed a quantitative assay for

their activities, and it was therefore impossible to detect and compare relative amounts of the factors during purification procedures. The major problem that had hindered efforts by previous investigators to characterize various factors had been the heterogeneous cultures of cells that had been used for the assays. Because of their heterogeneity, it was impossible to tell which of the cells were responding to which of the many factors in the lymphocyte-conditioned medium.

Because we had already established monoclonal lines of growth-factor–dependent cells, however, the problem of cell heterogeneity in the assay was solved. Also, as a postdoctoral fellow, I had developed a quantitative assay for erythropoietin, the red-blood-cell growth factor; it was relatively simple to adapt the method to measuring T cell growth factor.

Armed with a rapid and quantitative assay, we performed a series of experiments published in several papers between 1978 and 1983 that collectively described for the first time the biological and biochemical characteristics of the T cell growth factor now known as interleukin-2. These studies showed that the immune system, after it senses an antigen, transfers the control over the immune response from an antigen-regulated mechanism to a hormonelike regulatory system (see Figure 5.1).

The general mechanism works as follows: When an antigen is introduced into the body, it is ingested by macrophages (a class of scavenger cells) and B cells. These cells digest the antigen and present short segments of the antigen molecules on their cell surface. Most T cells in the body do not recognize the presented antigens, and they continue to move quietly through the bloodstream and lymphatic system. A few T cells, however, have antigen receptors that bind to the presented antigens, stimulating the cells. Thereafter, these antigen-stimulated T cells become autonomous growth-factor factories, both secreting IL-2 and responding to it by proliferating. The end result of this process is an expansion of only those T cell clones that react to the antigen stimulus.

Although we were able to demonstrate that only antigen-activated T cells responded to IL-2, we did not know how IL-2 interacted with the cells to produce its effects. I suspected that the mechanism would probably involve cell-surface receptors for IL-2, just as receptors for insulin mediate the activity of that hormone. Our experiments soon showed that activated T cells could absorb IL-2 activity, as

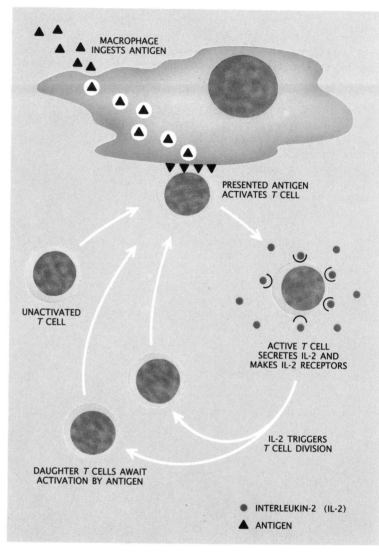

Figure 5.1 PROLIFERATION of *T* cells is controlled by IL-2 after an antigen, ingested and presented by a macrophage, activates individual *T* cells. The antigen stimulates the *T* cells to secrete IL-2 and to make IL-2 receptors. Subsequently, the binding of IL-2 to its receptors signals the *T* cells to divide, thereby producing pairs of daughter cells that can also be activated by the antigen. In this way, a clone of identical antigen-specific *T* cells grows until the immune system eliminates the antigen from the body.

would be expected if they bore IL-2 receptors. These findings encouraged us to produce and purify radioactively labeled IL-2, with which we could observe the process directly. The results from our very first experiments were unambiguous: IL-2 binds to cells because of a high-affinity receptor on the cell surface.

The application of this hormone-and-receptor concept to the immune system has had an extraordinary impact on models of immune regulation. Cellular immunology had previously maintained that

macrophages, *B* cells and *T* cells signaled one another exclusively through intimate contact. After the discovery of IL-2 and other soluble factors and the advent of the idea that the expression of IL-2 receptors determines which cells participate in the immune response, the interactions of the immune-system cells lost their mystical aura. It was possible to understand them according to principles borrowed from endocrinology—principles that describe the interactions of hormones and their receptors.

It was evident by 1982 that understanding the molecular mechanisms signaling *T* cells to proliferate was going to require a knowledge of the structures of IL-2 and its receptor. Structural knowledge would also be necessary to design agents that could therapeutically block or mimic the hormone-receptor interaction. An important first step toward these goals was the isolation of the gene for IL-2, which was first accomplished in 1983 by Tadatsugu Taniguchi and his colleagues at Tokyo University.

Once a gene has been isolated, gene-cloning technology makes it feasible to produce the gene's protein product in virtually unlimited quantities. In the past six years, IL-2 has been made available by biotechnology firms and distributed throughout the world. The availability of large quantities of pure IL-2 permitted David B. McKay and his group at the University of Colorado at Boulder to grow crystals of IL-2 and to deduce the three-dimensional structure of the molecule by X-ray crystallography in 1987 (see Figure 5.2).

In 1984 Warren J. Leonard and others, working in

Thomas A. Waldmann's laboratory at NCI, and Toshio Nikaido, working with Tasuku Honjo, Takashi Uchiyama and others at Kyoto University, simultaneously reported the isolation of a gene for a putative IL-2-receptor protein. This protein chain reacted with a monoclonal antibody against the IL-2 receptor developed by Uchiyama; however, the chain's small size and low affinity for IL-2 meant that it could not be the complete IL-2 receptor. Then, in 1986, Keisuke Teshigawara of Kyoto University, working in our laboratory at Dartmouth, and Mitsuru Tsudo, also of Kyoto University but working in Waldmann's laboratory, independently made the startling discovery of a second, larger IL-2 receptor chain.

It turned out that the IL-2 receptor is made up of two chains: one that is 55 kilodaltons in size and reacts with Uchiyama's antibody and an additional chain that is 75 kilodaltons in size. Michael Sharon of the National Institute of Child Health and Human Development, working with Leonard, also had data consistent with this interpretation. By the

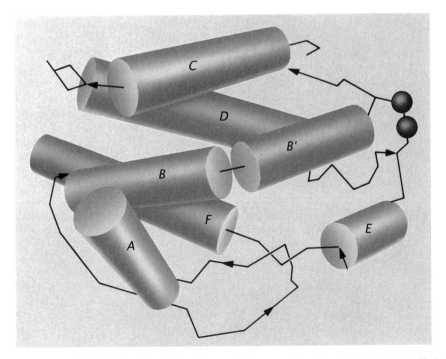

Figure 5.2 STRUCTURE of the IL-2 molecule has been revealed by X-ray crystallography. The 133 amino acids in the protein backbone of the molecule are coiled and folded into a roughly spherical shape; the cylinders (*A-F*) represent tight coils. The IL-2 molecule must be structurally intact to react with both protein chains in the IL-2 receptor.

fall of 1986 most workers in the field began to race toward the isolation and characterization of the new 75-kilodalton chain.

Tsudo eventually won this race after taking a new position in Tokyo at the Metropolitan Institute for Medical Sciences. By mid-1988 he had derived monoclonal antibodies that reacted with the 75-kilodalton chain. Subsequently, he collaborated with Masanori Hatakeyama, a young hematologist working in Taniguchi's laboratory at Osaka University. Using Tsudo's antibodies, Hatakeyama was able to identify and isolate the gene encoding the 75-kilodalton chain.

While these studies were proceeding, we devoted our efforts at Dartmouth to defining the role of the IL-2-receptor system in the immune response. In a series of experiments, Doreen A. Cantrell determined how the IL-2-receptor mechanism functions during a model T cell immune response. She discovered that there are only three parameters important for regulating T cell proliferation after antigen activation: the concentration of IL-2, the density of IL-2 receptors on the cell surface and the duration of the IL-2-receptor interaction. Apparently, before a cell will irrevocably commit to dividing, it must experience a number of IL-2-receptor interactions over several hours.

Huey-Mei Wang, a recent graduate student in my laboratory, extended these findings by showing that the IL-2 receptor functions as an "on-off" switch. IL-2 binds rapidly to the receptor by interacting with the binding site on the 55-kilodalton chain. It is then tightly held by an interaction with the binding site on the 75-kilodalton chain. (It is because IL-2 must interact with both receptor chains that the molecule must be intact to function.) This interaction between the IL-2 molecule and the 75-kilodalton chain turns on the intracellular mechanisms that signal the T cell to become active. When the molecule dissociates from the receptor, which happens only very slowly because of the strength of the interaction with the large chain, the signaling stops.

As the immune response proceeds, antigen gradually disappears from the body, and the antigen-reactive T cells stop receiving signals from their antigen receptors. Consequently, the number of IL-2 receptors on the cells gradually declines and the expanded clone of cells stops proliferating. These lingering T cells make up the memory population of the immune system.

T cells are not the only cells stimulated by IL-2. As early as 1981 Christopher S. Henney and his colleagues at the University of Washington reported that cells with natural killer (NK) activity are stimulated by IL-2. NK cells make up about 10 percent of the total circulating lymphocyte population and are thought to participate in the immune surveillance against cancer cells and in the body's initial responses to viruses; they may serve as a first line of defense by virtue of their immediate responsiveness to IL-2. Unlike T cells, NK cells have no antigen receptors and appear always to be in a state of activation. Studies have revealed that NK cells express the 75-kilodalton chain of the IL-2 receptor continuously.

B cells, like T cells, remain inactive until they make contact with antigen. They then undergo clonal expansion and become plasma cells, releasing large amounts of antibody. IL-2's role in these cellular changes is still somewhat controversial, but most investigators agree that it promotes the proliferation of antigen-activated B cell clones in the same way that it stimulates T cell growth. In addition, recent experiments by Marian E. Koshland of the University of California at Berkeley and Kenji Nakanishi from the Hyogo College of Medicine have demonstrated that IL-2 participates in the differentiation of B cells by helping them to start secreting antibodies.

All of these findings indicated that the IL-2-receptor mechanism plays a crucial role in regulating the first events of an immune response. It was therefore easy to imagine ways of exploiting this hormone-receptor interaction either to enhance or to suppress the immune response for therapeutic purposes. Actually, the two most effective types of immunosuppressive drugs prescribed today, cyclosporine and the glucocorticoids, turned out to work by inhibiting the production of IL-2.

My colleague Thomas L. Ciardelli of Dartmouth hopes to capitalize on the IL-2-receptor system by creating modified forms of the IL-2 molecule that could serve either as IL-2 antagonists (by tying up the receptor without activating it) or as "superleukins" with greater immunostimulatory effects. A similarly imaginative approach to immunosuppression has been developed independently by John R. Murphy of Boston University and Ira H. Pastan of NCI. With genetic-engineering techniques, these investigators have coupled bacterial toxins to IL-2. These toxic hybrid molecules bind to and kill antigen-activated T cells and B cells, thereby deleting an antigen-specific clone from the body (see Figure 5.3).

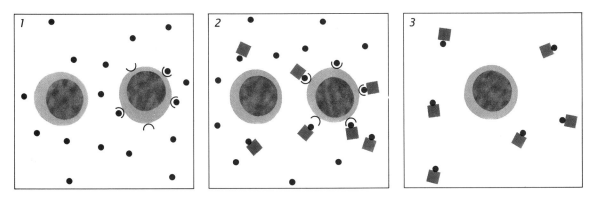

• IL-2
▪ IL-2 CONJUGATED TO TOXIN

Figure 5.3 DELETING a specific clone of *T* cells is a route to suppressing the immune system selectively. One way to do so would be to administer IL-2 conjugated to a bacterial toxin. Only *T* cells that have been activated by antigen make IL-2 and IL-2 receptors (*1*). Hence, the IL-2 toxin conjugate would bind with and kill only the active *T* cells (*2*). The inactive *T* cells would not be harmed by the conjugate molecules (*3*).

Monoclonal antibodies that react with IL-2 or its receptor can also suppress antigen-activated *T* cell responses. Antibodies that block the binding of IL-2 to its receptor completely inhibit the antigen-specific proliferation of *T* cells in culture; the antibodies have also proved to be effective antigen-specific immunosuppressants in heart-transplantation experiments. The same function might be served by a different preparation, consisting of the IL-2-binding portion of the receptor molecules, which could compete with cell-surface receptors for IL-2 (see Figure 5.4).

IL-2 itself has several obvious applications as an immune stimulant. Because IL-2 stimulates the clonal expansion of *T* cells and *B* cells after the introduction of antigen, one obvious use for IL-2

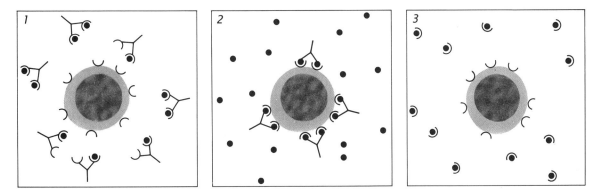

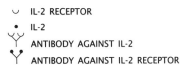

⌣ IL-2 RECEPTOR
• IL-2
Y IL-2 ANTIBODY AGAINST IL-2
Y ANTIBODY AGAINST IL-2 RECEPTOR

Figure 5.4 SELECTIVE SUPPRESSION of the immune response would be desirable for treating organ-transplant patients and people with autoimmune diseases. One approach might be to interfere with the binding between IL-2 molecules and their receptors on *T* cells, for example, by injecting antibodies against IL-2 into the body (*1*). Antibodies against the IL-2 receptor should have the same effect, because the IL-2 molecules would be unable to find unoccupied receptors (*2*). Another possibility would involve injected soluble IL-2 receptors, which could compete with the cellular receptors (*3*).

will be as an immunopotentiator: a substance that boosts the effectiveness of vaccinations. The safety and efficacy of IL-2 has already been tested in human beings by Stefan C. Meuer of the University of Heidelberg during immunization trials with a hepatitis B vaccine. As additional vaccines are developed by genetic engineering, the availability of an effective immunostimulator such as IL-2 may well determine their eventual success or failure.

IL-2 has already been applied as an experimental immunotherapy for cancer. Pioneered by Steven A. Rosenberg and his colleagues at NCI, this strategy culminates an almost century-long search for an effective way of harnessing the immune system to destroy cancer cells. So far, patients with at least three types of cancers that are usually extremely resistant to conventional therapies—malignant melanoma, kidney cancer and colon cancer—have responded to the administration of IL-2 in combination with IL-2-stimulated NK cells. The proportion of patients that have had a significant response to therapy is still low, about 20 percent. Yet many of the patients who have responded have had remarkably stable, disease-free remissions without any further therapy.

One of the most promising areas for immunoenhancement therapy lies in the treatment of infectious diseases. Since the introduction of antibiotics in the late 1940's and 1950's, most of the developed world has been relatively free of the most common bacterial diseases. Equally effective antimicrobial agents against fungi, parasites and viruses have not yet been developed, however. Moreover, infectious diseases continue to be major health problems in developing countries.

Many chronic infectious diseases that do not respond to conventional treatments, such as tuberculosis, leprosy and leishmaniasis, involve microbial infestations of macrophages. These infected macrophages steadily release inflammatory substances that can eventually destroy the surrounding tissues. From results obtained by Gilla Kaplan, Zanvil A. Cohn and their colleagues at the Rockefeller University, it now seems that the activation and expansion of T cells and NK cells by IL-2 can tip the scales in the favor of the immune system: IL-2-stimulated cells can kill the infected cells and the microbes they contain. The Third World could be the first place to benefit from such immunotherapy.

AIDS shares many features of these other chronic infectious diseases. The human immunodeficiency virus (HIV), however, infects helper T cells as well as macrophages, with the result that patients eventually lose the very cells that are critical for mounting an effective immune response. Consequently, people with AIDS become susceptible to any and all the common microbes in the environment. Investigators are now beginning clinical trials of IL-2 for the treatment of HIV infection, administering it before the overt immunodeficiency develops. If HIV-infected cells can be killed by IL-2-activated T cells and NK cells before the virus becomes widespread, patients may be spared the devastating loss of their immune cells.

The converse goal of immunosuppression is important primarily in developed countries, where organ transplants and autoimmune diseases are more common. The currently available drugs are broadly immunosuppressive and must be taken over long periods; consequently, organ-transplant recipients and patients with autoimmune diseases run serious risks of potentially fatal infections during treatment. An approach is needed that, for example, suppresses only those immune cells reactive to a grafted organ or tissue while sparing the rest of the immune cells. Any approach that capitalizes on the blocking of the IL-2-receptor interaction will provide that much-needed specificity.

In the 30 years since Burnet first enunciated the clonal-selection theory, a detailed cellular and molecular understanding has been crafted that explains how the immune system is regulated. The appreciation of the fundamental role of IL-2 in mediating the expansion of a clone of immune cells after it has been selected by an antigen has been instrumental to this understanding. New means of stimulating or suppressing the immune system for the treatment of diseases can now be created based on a rational understanding of immunity.

Tumor Necrosis Factor

First identified because of its anticancer activity, the factor is now recognized to be one of a family of proteins that orchestrate the body's remarkably complex response to injury and infection.

· · ·

Lloyd J. Old
May, 1988

Rare events, properly interpreted, have been the source of much progress in science. The spontaneous regression of cancer is a case in point. Before the turn of the century a few astute physicians observed that shrinkage of malignant tumors in patients sometimes coincided with the development of bacterial infections. They postulated that infectious agents or their products might somehow fight cancer.

This notion, and the later data that supported it, prompted decades of search for a mechanism that could lead from infection to cancer regression. Some evidence suggested that the bacteria did not kill tumors directly but instead strengthened the activity of forces in the body that are capable of restraining cancer. In pursuit of this idea, my colleagues and I at the Memorial Sloan-Kettering Cancer Center some 15 years ago discovered a small polypeptide, or protein, that is produced by the body in the course of bacterial infections and that kills tumors in mice. We and others are now in the early stages of testing the substance, which we named tumor necrosis factor, as an anticancer treatment for human beings.

Although the factor was initially discovered because of its cancer-killing activity, efforts to eluci-

date its functions further have revealed that it is also a central regulator of inflammation and immunity, the intertwined processes that limit and repair injuries and fight infection. It is one of a family of so-called cytokines: polypeptide mediators that transmit signals from one cell to another. Together with other substances, cytokines constitute the molecular language of inflammation and immunity and form a complex interacting and overlapping network of signals that orchestrate the body's defensive reactions. These potent and sometimes toxic proteins can elicit, enhance or inhibit one another's effects.

Like tumor necrosis factor, certain other cytokines, such as interferon (a general term for several structurally related molecules), are known to have anticancer activity and are also showing some promise as cancer therapies. A gradually deepening understanding of the individual and combined effects of the cytokines is leading to treatments for other conditions as well. For example, interferon has been shown in human trials to control certain viral infections; other cytokines that stimulate the production of infection-fighting blood cells are also being tested in the clinic. It seems likely that cytokines themselves, or substances that induce their

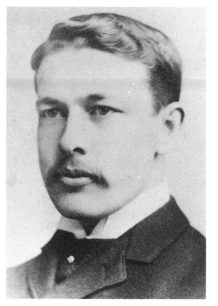

Figure 6.1 WILLIAM B. COLEY stimulated much of the research that led to the discovery of tumor necrosis factor. Near the turn of this century he began to treat cancer patients with a killed-bacteria vaccine and observed that their tumors sometimes regressed. Later work showed that the vaccine did not kill cancers in the test tube, a finding that provoked a search for latent anticancer forces aroused in the body by bacterial products. The search resulted in the identification of TNF in the 1970's.

release, will eventually be administered to strengthen the body's ability to fight a wide range of diseases. Conversely, inhibitory factors that restrain the polypeptide mediators in instances where they are toxic are also likely to become valuable therapeutic agents.

The story of the discovery of tumor necrosis factor properly begins with William B. Coley, a surgeon at Memorial Hospital in New York from 1892 to 1931 (see Figure 6.1). In the late 19th century he and a few other physicians had some success in treating cancer patients by infecting them with liver bacteria. There were, however, serious problems with this approach. Infection could not be induced in some patients. Moreover, in the pre-antibiotic era the difficulty of controlling the infections that did result was cause for concern. Coley therefore developed vaccines of killed bacteria, which came to be known as Coley's toxins. These reproduced many of the symptoms of bacterial infection, such as fever and chills, but they could be administered without fear of producing an actual infection. Tumors in some patients treated with the toxins diminished or disappeared, but (as was the case with infection by live bacteria) the results were inconsistent. In the end radiation therapy and chemotherapy essentially supplanted Coley's approach.

Interest in the potential value of microbes as treatments for cancer might have died with Coley, but his daughter Helen Coley Nauts of the Cancer Research Institute dedicated herself to making physicians aware of his results. Interest also lived on in the laboratory. There investigators confirmed that a range of infectious agents and their products had anticancer effects in animals. In particular, they demonstrated that the injection of live or killed strains of gram-negative bacteria could cause hemorrhagic necrosis of mouse tumors: the tumors bled into themselves, turned black and dried up (see Figure 6.2).

In work that was important to the later discovery of tumor necrosis factor, Murray J. Shear and his colleagues at the National Cancer Institute in 1943 identified and purified the active component of the gram-negative bacteria, determining that it was a complex fat-and-sugar compound now called lipopolysaccharide (LPS). Subsequent work showed that the compound is a constituent of the bacteria's outer wall and that it has both beneficial and harmful effects. In addition to causing hemorrhagic necrosis of tumors, LPS increases an animal's resistance to new bacterial infections and to lethal doses of X rays. In minute quantities the substance also causes fever, which in moderation may well help to combat infection; in greater amounts LPS can lead to

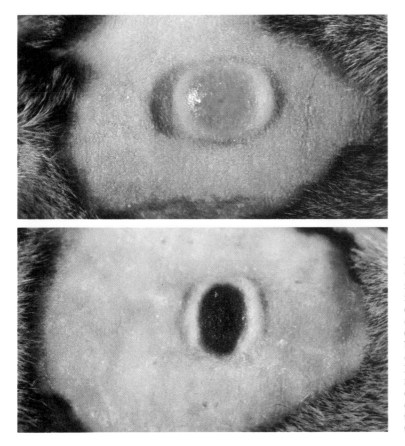

Figure 6.2 HEMORRHAGIC NE-CROSIS of a cancerous tumor in a mouse occurs soon after the animal is injected with endotoxin, a component of gram-negative bacteria. Whereas the cancer in an untreated animal thrives (*top*), the tumor in the treated animal bleeds into itself (hence the black color) and dies (*bottom*). It is now believed that this effect of endotoxin is not a direct one. Instead the endotoxin causes certain cells in the body to secrete tumor necrosis factor (TNF), which then acts as an agent of tumor destruction.

shock and death. (The toxic properties of LPS account for its other name, endotoxin.)

In the late 1950's Baruj Benacerraf, then at the New York University Medical Center, and I studied another bacterial agent that later would also play a role in the discovery of tumor necrosis factor: bacillus Calmette-Guérin, or BCG. This microbe, an attenuated form of the organism causing tuberculosis, induces a self-limiting infection in mice and makes them more resistant to subsequent bacterial infection and to tumor growth.

These animal studies and others demonstrated that bacterial products could indeed lead to the destruction of cancers, but the findings by no means explained how they did so. Test-tube studies provided a hint: neither LPS nor BCG inhibited or killed tumor cells directly. Surely the microbial action was indirect and was mediated by something in the host. It was at this stage that Elizabeth A. Carswell, Rob-

ert L. Kassel, Barbara D. Williamson and I discovered tumor necrosis factor.

While searching for substances produced by the body that would restrain the growth of cancer and yet leave normal cells unharmed, we had noted that blood drawn from normal mice inhibited the growth of leukemic cells in other mice while exerting no apparent effect on their healthy tissues. Now we wanted to find ways to increase the level of the putative cancer-inhibiting factor. Since LPS and BCG render mice more resistant to tumor growth, we injected these substances into healthy mice, drew blood and examined the effect of the blood on tumors in other mice.

In one set of tests we injected animals with BCG and, some days later, injected them with LPS. Blood from these mice induced hemorrhagic necrosis in tumors of other animals and was highly toxic to cancer cells in the test tube. After ruling out the possibility that residual BCG and residual LPS (a more difficult possibility to exclude) in the blood might have been responsible for the tumor damage in the treated mice, we were left with one probable explanation for our findings: the animals injected with BCG and LPS had produced large amounts of an antitumor factor, and it was this factor that was responsible for the cancer killing. In view of the striking damage the substance did to mouse tumors, we called it tumor necrosis factor. The factor has subsequently been found to reproduce—and to be a mediator of—many of the effects of BCG and LPS.

What was the source of tumor necrosis factor? For several reasons we assumed it came mainly from activated macrophages, or cells that engulf and degrade bacteria, dead cells and other debris in the body (see Figure 6.3). In particular, we knew that both BCG and LPS activate macrophages and increase their number in the body, and we knew that when macrophages stimulated by LPS or BCG are mixed with tumor cells, the tumor cells are killed.

Once we discovered tumor necrosis factor in mice, we quickly showed that rabbits, rats and guinea pigs also produce it. The next step was to isolate it from blood serum and define its chemical characteristics so that enough of it could be produced for extensive study. The process of purifica-

tion was arduous because, although the factor can be detected in blood drawn from animals treated with BCG and LPS, it is usually present in extremely small amounts. Moreover, at each stage of purification we had to satisfy ourselves that the factor was still present. We did so by assaying each isolate for specified activities. For example, the isolate had to cause hemorrhagic necrosis of tumors in animals; it had to kill certain types of cancer cells in the test tube, and the effect had to be produced by progressively smaller quantities at successive stages of purification.

Saul Green, a colleague of ours at Sloan-Kettering, began the purification process and isolated enough of the mouse factor to enable us to demonstrate that the effect on animal tumors and the effect on malignant cells in the test tube were the work of a single substance rather than of two associated substances, one active in the body and the other active in the test tube. We also demonstrated that the substance is a protein. Katsuyuki Haranaka, first as a member of our group and then with Nobuko Satomi of the University of Tokyo, continued the effort and eventually succeeded in obtaining a single polypeptide—pure tumor necrosis factor—from the blood of both mice and rabbits.

Meanwhile Danielle N. Männel and Stephan E.

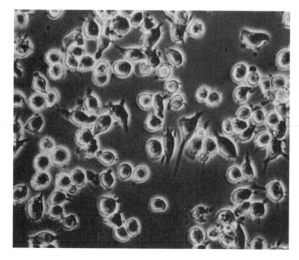 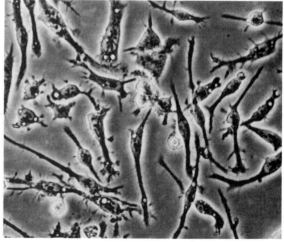

Figure 6.3 MACROPHAGES (*left*) spread and enlarge (*right*) when they are exposed to LPS, indicating that they have become activated. The cells, which play a central role in inflammation and immunity and can kill cancer cells, secrete dozens of factors, including tumor necrosis factor, that carry out many of their activities. For example, Hans Schreiber and his colleagues at the University of Chicago and Genentech, Inc., have shown that TNF is an important mediator of cancer-cell killing by activated macrophages.

Mergenhagen of the National Institute of Dental Research and N. Matthews of the University of Wales proved that macrophages do indeed produce tumor necrosis factor. In search of a human cell type that could be coaxed to produce high quantities of the factor in culture, Williamson, Carswell and I, along with Berish Y. Rubin of the New York Blood Center, then screened many types of human cells and found that defensive cells other than macrophages also secreted a factor that exhibited the known activities of tumor necrosis factor.

Our work with the mouse and human factors soon enabled us to uncover two features of tumor necrosis factor that may have important implications for treatment. We found that tumor necrosis factor and interferon—which was also known to have antitumor effects—act synergistically. Exposure of cancerous cells to both factors together results in a far greater cell kill than would be expected if the individual effects of the two substances were simply added together. We also found that human tumor necrosis factor, like the mouse variety, lacks species specificity: it kills cancer cells from mice as well as from human beings. Interferon, in contrast, is species-specific.

The decade-long effort to purify tumor necrosis factor finally culminated in 1984 with the cloning of the gene, the identification of the protein's amino acid sequence and the production of large quantities of the factor by several groups associated with biotechnology companies, including David V. Goeddel and his colleagues at Genentech, Inc., and Walter Fiers and his co-workers at the State University of Ghent and at Biogen SA (see Figure 6.4). Since then there has been an explosion of information about the factor's activities.

It is now clear that tumor necrosis factor elicits a remarkable range of reactions in the body and that it will be some time before a complete picture of its normal functions is constructed. Nevertheless, research has shown that tumor necrosis factor is crucial to inflammation and immunity, is secreted early in these processes and stimulates defensive cells to produce many other polypeptides.

In order to understand the role of tumor necrosis factor in inflammation and immunity, one must have a sense of the events set in motion by an injury, whether it results from mechanical trauma, from chemicals or from infection. What follows is a highly simplified outline and necessarily omits a host of important actors and events. I should point out that, in theory, inflammation can be viewed as the aspect of the defensive function that confines and repairs injury, and immunity as the aspect that specifically neutralizes invading microbes and confers specific resistance to future infection by the same invader. In reality the two are inseparable: most of the cells and molecules that defend the body are involved in both inflammation and immunity.

In the first phase of the response to injury white blood cells known as polymorphonuclear leukocytes, or granulocytes, leave the flowing blood and adhere to endothelial cells, the cells that line blood vessels (see Figure 6.5). The endothelial cells spread apart somewhat and enable the granulocytes to pass into the injured tissue, where they ingest and destroy any microbes that may have entered the wound. (When large numbers of the white cells accumulate and die at the inflamed site, they form pus.)

Macrophages soon join the battle in force and replace the granulocytes as the predominant cell type at the injury. The macrophages swallow and destroy bacteria, particularly those coated with antibody, and damaged cells. At the same time other blood cells also become more active: T lymphocytes (white cells that mature in the thymus) proliferate and arouse other defensive cells, including B lymphocytes, which divide, differentiate and secrete antibodies in quantity. As the infection is controlled, connective-tissue cells called fibroblasts and other cells begin to repair damaged tissue.

Tumor necrosis factor starts to exert its many effects once macrophages, which also release the cytokines known as interleukin-1 and colony-stimulating factors, take the offensive. Interleukin-1 is unlike tumor necrosis factor in structure but has many of the same activities. Colony-stimulating factors cause the bone marrow to produce blood cells, such as polymorphonuclear leukocytes and monocytes (which are precursors of macrophages).

Michael P. Bevilacqua, Jordan S. Pober and Michael A. Gimbrone, Jr., of the Harvard Medical School have found that both tumor necrosis factor and interleukin-1 stimulate endothelial cells to synthesize molecules that increase the adhesion of granulocytes to the surface of blood vessels. Tumor necrosis factor also has a direct effect on the granulocytes, increasing their attachment to the vessel wall and their migration into damaged tissue. In addition, Michael A. Palladino, Jr., of Genentech and Carl F. Nathan of the Cornell University Medi-

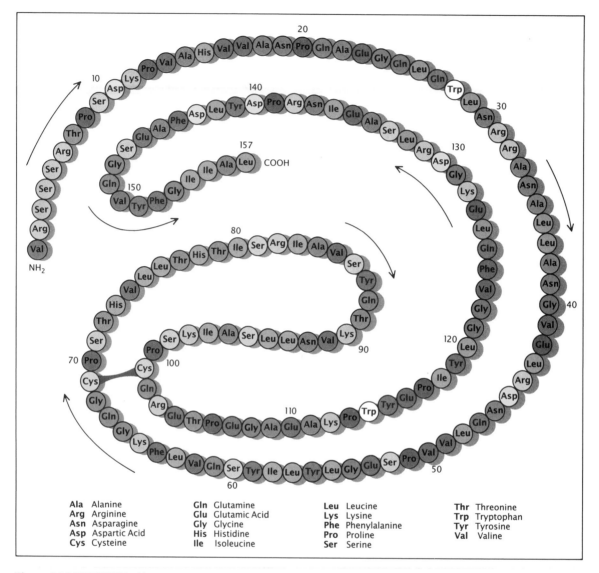

Ala	Alanine	Gln	Glutamine	Leu	Leucine	Thr	Threonine
Arg	Arginine	Glu	Glutamic Acid	Lys	Lysine	Trp	Tryptophan
Asn	Asparagine	Gly	Glycine	Phe	Phenylalanine	Tyr	Tyrosine
Asp	Aspartic Acid	His	Histidine	Pro	Proline	Val	Valine
Cys	Cysteine	Ile	Isoleucine	Ser	Serine		

Figure 6.4 MOLECULE of human tumor necrosis factor is a protein consisting of 157 amino acids. The amino acid sequence was determined in 1984, the year the gene encoding TNF was first cloned by several groups associated with biotechnology companies.

cal College have demonstrated that the factor is one of the most potent signals for stimulating granulocytes to produce toxic oxygen products that destroy bacteria.

Tumor necrosis factor, along with interleukin-1, also plays a part in the activation of *T* lymphocytes. These cells in turn produce interleukin-2 (a growth factor for *T* and *B* cells), gamma interferon (which further activates macrophages), several other factors that trigger the multiplication of *B* cells, and colony-stimulating factors (see Figure 6.6). Activated *T* cells produce a substance known as lymphotoxin as well; this cytokine is quite similar to tumor necrosis factor in both structure and function. It was discovered by Gale A. Granger and T. W. Williams of the University of California at Irvine and Nancy H. Ruddle

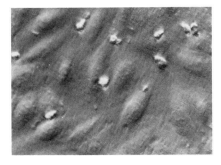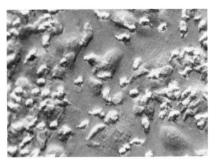

Figure 6.5 ONE ACTIVITY of tumor necrosis factor can be demonstrated readily in the test tube. Endothelial cells (*large bumps*), which line blood vessels, do not ordinarily interact with polymorphonuclear leukocytes (*bright bodies*)—a type of white blood cell that digests bacteria—when the cells are mixed (*left*). Exposure of the endothelial cells to TNF or interleukin-1 causes the cells to synthesize molecules that promote the adherence of leukocytes (*right*). A similar phenomenon presumably occurs in the body: in response to an injury, TNF and other factors promote the attachment of leukocytes to the blood-vessel wall, aiding their migration into injured tissue.

and Byron H. Waksman of the Yale University School of Medicine.

Like the *T* lymphocytes, *B* lymphocytes are affected by tumor necrosis factor and interleukin-1. The factors regulate the production of antibodies by *B* cells; they also cause many cell types, including endothelial cells and fibroblasts, to secrete still more of the colony-stimulating factors.

Certain systemic effects of the inflammatory and immune responses can also be traced in part to tumor necrosis factor and other cytokines. For instance, tumor necrosis factor and interleukin-1 act on the temperature centers of the brain to produce fever. Another effect—the increased circulation in the blood of so-called acute-phase proteins—is an indirect result of the release of tumor necrosis factor. The acute-phase proteins, produced by the liver, are thought to increase the efficiency of inflammatory reactions, and they appear to be regulated by a recently described factor called interleukin-6. This factor is synthesized by a variety of cell types in response to tumor necrosis factor, interleukin-1 or interferon.

Inflammation and immunity, like all other normal reactions of the body, are meant to preserve or restore health. They can nonetheless cause a range of uncomfortable symptoms. The typical effects were identified by the Roman physician Aulus Cornelius Celsus: *rubor* (redness), *tumor* (swelling), *calor* (heat) and *dolor* (pain). Symptoms can vary widely, however, and include such discomforts as the stuffy, runny nose of a cold or an allergy. It gener-

ally is not the microbes invading the body that make one feel ill but the body's response to those invaders. If the defensive response is too vigorous or goes on too long—as it does when an infection is chronic—it can actually do permanent harm. Such is the case with rheumatoid arthritis, in which chronic inflammation can produce debilitating effects. A vigorous inflammatory response can also cause shock and death. Recent work implicates tumor necrosis factor as a cause of many negative effects associated with the defensive response.

For instance, studies have suggested that tumor necrosis factor might contribute to cachexia: a condition marked by a profound weight loss stemming from the disappearance of fat deposits and the shrinkage of muscles. This disorder sometimes develops when the body fails to overcome an infection; it is also observed in some patients with cancer.

Several years ago Bruce Beutler and Anthony Cerami of Rockefeller University found that a factor produced by activated macrophages inhibits an enzyme, lipoprotein lipase, that is crucial for the normal storage of fat and is suppressed in cachectic individuals. When the factor, which the workers called cachectin, was purified and its amino acid sequence determined, it was found to be identical with tumor necrosis factor. Subsequent work showed that interleukin-1 and interferon also inhibit lipoprotein lipase activity in the test tube. The role of these three cytokines and other factors in causing cachexia in patients with chronic infection or cancer needs further definition.

FAMILY	MEMBERS	OTHER NAMES
Interferons (IFN)	IFN-α	Leukocyte Interferon
	IFN-β	Fibroblast Interferon
	IFN-γ	Immune Interferon
Tumor Necrosis Factors (TNF)	TNF	TNF-α, Cachectin
	Lymphotoxin	TNF-β
Interleukins (IL)	IL-1 α, IL-1 β	Endogenous Pyrogen, Lymphocyte-Activating Factor, Leukocyte Endogenous Mediator, Hemopoietin 1
	IL-2	T-Cell Growth Factor
	IL-3	Multipotential CSF, Mast Cell Growth Factor
	IL-4	B-Cell Stimulatory Factor 1 (BSF-1)
	IL-5	T-Cell Replacing Factor (TRF), Eosinophil Differentiation Factor, B-Cell Growth Factor-II (BCGF-II)
	IL-6	B-Cell Stimulatory Factor 2 (BSF-2), Interferon-β$_2$ Hepatocyte-Stimulating Factor (HSF)
Colony-Stimulating Factors (CSF)	Granulocyte Macrophage-CSF (GM-CSF)	CSF-2
	Granulocyte-CSF (G-CSF)	Pluripoietin
	Macrophage-CSF (M-CSF)	CSF-1
	Erythropoietin	
Other Growth and Regulatory Factors (GF)	Epidermal Growth Factor (EGF)	
	Fibroblast Growth Factor (Acidic- and Basic-FGF)	
	Insulin-like Growth Factor-1 (IGF-1)	Somatomedin C
	Insulin-like Growth Factor-2 (IGF-2)	Somatomedin A
	Nerve Growth Factor (NGF)	
	Platelet-Derived Growth Factor (PDGF)	
	Transforming Growth Factor-α (TGF-α)	
	Transforming Growth Factor-β (TGF-β)	

Figure 6.6 PROTEIN FACTORS involved in inflammation, immunity and the growth and inhibition of cells are often grouped into families. There is considerable overlap in the activities of the factors, however: structurally unrelated molecules, such as tumor necrosis factor and interleukin-1, elicit many of the same effects. Adding to the complexity, individual factors can cause cells to secrete other factors and can potentiate or antagonize one another's effects. Lymphotoxin is produced by T lymphocytes. It is grouped with TNF because it is structurally and functionally related to the TNF produced by macrophages.

Investigations into the ability of tumor necrosis factor to mediate the effects of LPS provided other indications of the factor's ability to do ill as well as good. Injection of large amounts of tumor necrosis factor in mice and other animals has been found to cause tissue injury, shock and death, just as LPS does. Yet at lower doses the factor exhibits the protective activities associated with low doses of LPS: it protects mice against bacterial infections, lethal doses of X rays and tumor growth.

Studies of parasitic diseases in animals have also been revealing. On the one hand, mice injected with tumor necrosis factor are more resistant to certain forms of malaria, and the factor has been shown to stimulate macrophages and other blood cells to kill the parasites that cause Chagas' disease and schistosomiasis. On the other hand, Pierre Vassalli and his colleagues at the University of Geneva have recently shown that the substance has a role in the death of mice with malaria that has invaded the brain: it appears to mediate a lethal inflammation of the brain tissue. The mice do not die if they receive an antibody that neutralizes the brain-damaging effect of tumor necrosis factor.

Another indication of the potential toxicity of tumor necrosis factor comes from human beings. A. Waage of the University of Trondheim in Norway has discovered that patients with severe meningococcal infections who have relatively high levels of the factor in their blood are more likely to die from shock than patients who have no detectable levels of the polypeptide.

With tumor necrosis factor as with many other factors produced by the body, there seems to be a fine line between benefit and harm: an agent that is helpful in the local control of injury and infection may be toxic when it is released in large amounts or in the wrong place. The growing awareness of the harmful potential of tumor necrosis factor has given rise to interest in the design of drugs that will block its action when its detrimental effects outweigh its protective ones.

In spite of the rapid accumulation of new information about tumor necrosis factor, my colleagues and I still do not fully understand how it causes the effects for which it was named: hemorrhage and necrosis of tumors. One partial explanation has to do with the factor's directive role in inflammation and immunity. Even if tumor necrosis factor were not directly toxic to tumors, the *T* cells and other cells it stimulates and the other cytokines those cells secrete when they are activated do sometimes join forces to destroy tumors.

Beyond this generalized antitumor role, however, there is clear evidence that tumor necrosis factor has a more immediate effect on cancer. In animal studies it has been shown to damage the blood vessels that nourish tumors. This damage reduces the flow of blood and oxygen to the tumor cells, which then starve and die (see Figure 6.7).

In contrast, it appears that in noncancerous tissue the cytokine actually plays an important role in normal angiogenesis (the formation of new blood vessels during development or growth, or the replacement of injured vessels in existing tissue). Marijke Fràter-Schröder of the University of Zurich and S. Joseph Leibovich of Northwestern University and their co-workers have demonstrated that injection of tumor necrosis factor into an animal induces normal endothelial cells to grow and join together to form new vessels. Tumor necrosis factor is not alone in exhibiting angiogenic activity; four other cytokines do the same. Nature, it seems, has chosen not to construct a different mediator or set of mediators for every process in the body but rather to call on the same molecules repeatedly for quite different purposes.

Why would blood vessels in a tumor respond to tumor necrosis factor so differently from those in normal organs? Investigators need to learn more about the regulation of angiogenesis before the question can be answered. One idea holds that tumor cells themselves, or defensive cells attracted to the tumor, may produce some factor that renders the tumor vessels susceptible to damage induced by tumor necrosis factor.

In addition to damaging a tumor's blood vessels,

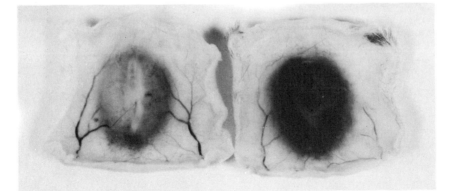

Figure 6.7 TINY BLOOD VESSELS normally feed a tumor (*left*), but the vessels inside the tumor are destroyed (*right*) and bleed within hours after a mouse is injected with tumor necrosis factor. Because such selective vascular damage deprives a tumor of oxygen and nutrients, most of its cells soon die. Much evidence suggests that vascular destruction is the major way TNF leads to hemorrhagic necrosis of tumors.

tumor necrosis factor in the body might also kill cancer cells directly, as it has long been known to do in the test tube. In one survey of cells from more than 60 different human cancers, my colleagues and I demonstrated three distinct responses to the factor: cell death, inhibition of cell growth and no effect. Approximately one-third of the tested cells fell into each category. Cells from breast cancer appeared to be most sensitive to the killing action of tumor necrosis factor, whereas cells from melanoma (a type of skin cancer) responded to the substance by growing at a reduced rate (see Figure 6.8). We also tested normal cells and found no inhibitory effect. In fact, Jan T. Vilček of the New York University School of Medicine has demonstrated that tumor necrosis factor actually stimulates cultured fibroblasts to grow more vigorously.

Because the first step in the action of many substances that influence cell activity is binding to specific receptors on the surface of the cell, Rubin, Vilček and others have independently looked to see whether the differential responses of cancer cells to tumor necrosis factor could be correlated with the presence or absence of receptors for the polypeptide. They did find factor-specific receptors but detected no relation between the number of receptors and the cells' responsiveness to tumor necrosis factor. Characteristics other than the number of receptors, then, must determine what the response to bound tumor necrosis factor will be.

One characteristic that might make a cell particularly sensitive to the toxicity of tumor necrosis factor is a reduced ability to repair damage caused by the factor. When George E. Gifford of the University of

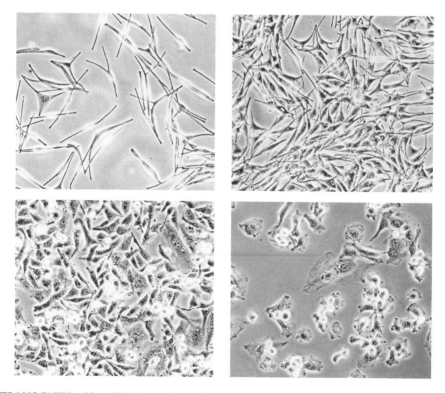

Figure 6.8 MELANOCYTES, skin cells that produce the pigment melanin (*top left*), proliferate markedly when exposed to tumor necrosis factor in the test tube (*top right*). In contrast, cells from melanoma, a skin cancer (*bottom left*), stop growing after exposure to TNF (*bottom right*), as Yuko Arita and Magdalena Eisinger of the Memorial Sloan-Kettering Cancer Center have shown. Such findings indicate that in addition to damaging tumor blood vessels, TNF might exert a direct, selective toxicity on cancer cells in the body.

Florida College of Medicine exposed cells to agents that inhibited their essential functions, such as the synthesis of RNA, he greatly enhanced the sensitivity of the cells to the toxic effects of tumor necrosis factor; even cells that would ordinarily not be affected could be killed. These results imply that cells do have a mechanism for repairing injury caused by tumor necrosis factor and that when the mechanism is absent (as it may be in certain cancer cells) or compromised (as it apparently was by Gifford's agents), cells exposed to tumor necrosis factor die. What actually causes the cell death is not known, but there is evidence that the cytokine activates intracellular enzymes that liberate highly reactive molecules. It may be the action of these molecules that injures and finally kills cancer cells.

A major goal of the extensive current research into the activities of tumor necrosis factor is the development of treatments for cancer. Preliminary clinical trials of the factor are now under way at many medical centers around the world. When the polypeptide has been administered so that it circulates throughout the body, only a few patients have had tumor inhibition at the doses studied to date. In Japan and Germany the factor has been injected directly into cancers. A number of the patients in those trials have had tumor regression, in some instances complete. There are side effects. Like other cytokines under study as cancer treatments, tumor necrosis factor can cause fever, chills, lethargy and a drop in blood pressure. Many patients feel as if they have come down with the flu.

Although clinical trials of tumor necrosis factor and other individual cytokines are aimed at revealing what each substance can do by itself, it seems likely that combinations of cytokines, or of cytokines with other substances, will be needed in order to produce the most successful cancer treatments. Indeed, on the basis of the fact that tumor necrosis factor and interferon act synergistically, Janice L. Gabrilove and Herbert F. Oettgen of Sloan-Kettering are now testing a therapy that couples these two agents (see Figure 6.9).

One of the preliminary findings is that certain doses of the combined agents cause patients to have sharp pain at the tumor site, where there had been no pain before. We do not yet know the cause, but such acute pain is suggestive of damage to blood vessels. We are now exploring the possibility that the treatment is damaging the blood vessels that feed the tumors. A number of other trials of combination therapies are planned as well: tumor necrosis factor will be paired with interleukin-2 (which has promise as an anticancer agent), chemotherapeutic agents, monoclonal antibodies or radiation.

Studies have now confirmed that William Coley's decision to treat cancer patients with microbes made good sense; when his toxins were successful, they almost certainly induced macrophages in the human body to produce tumor necrosis factor and other factors that in combination exerted anticancer effects. Why then has Coley's approach been ignored by most clinicians for so many years?

For one thing, an understanding of how the toxins worked required an understanding of inflammation and immunity; it has only been in recent

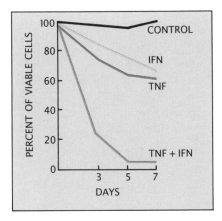

Figure 6.9 INTERFERON AND TNF have a synergistic effect on human breast-cancer cells. When the factors are mixed together, they destroy more malignant cells (*orange*) than would be killed if the independent effects of the interferon (*yellow*) and the TNF (*red*) were added together. Such synergy indicates that cancer treatments combining the two substances will probably prove more effective than therapies consisting of either substance alone.

years that critical molecules involved in these processes have been identified and isolated. In addition, the response to Coley's toxins varied widely from patient to patient, with many people not benefiting at all.

From our current perspective it seems likely that patients who did not respond may have been unable to produce tumor necrosis factor or the other cytokines that activate inflammation and immunity and are destructive to cancer. Now that tumor necrosis factor and many of the other factors elicited in the course of infection have been identified, it may be possible to employ them as new, more effective versions of Coley's toxins.

We are just beginning. If we are fortunate, the new treatments will consistently arouse the body's natural anticancer forces and produce the tumor regressions that have fueled the imagination of generations of cancer researchers. The forces exist; the task ahead is to find ways to unleash them.

How Killer Cells Kill

These immune-system cells recognize a target, close in on it and bind tightly to it. Then they secrete onto its surface a lethal pore-forming protein that causes the target cell to leak and die.

. . .

John Ding-E Young and Zanvil A. Cohn
January, 1988

The immune system is commonly likened to an army and its various cells to soldiers. The analogy is nowhere more appropriate than in the case of the cells called killer cells. Their primary duty is to seek out and destroy the body's own cells when they go wrong: to kill tumor cells and cells that have been infected by viruses (and perhaps by other foreign agents). For some years it has been clear that killer cells do their job with great efficiency, first seeking out a miscreant target cell, then binding tightly to it and finally doing something to it that causes its death, while at the same time sparing innocent bystander cells. But what exactly do they do? Just how do the killer cells kill?

The answer is beginning to come clear. Having bound to an appropriate victim, the killer cell takes aim at the target's surface and shoots it full of holes (see Figure 7.1). More specifically, it fires molecules of a lethal protein. The molecules bore into the target cell's surface membrane and form porelike channels. The target cell leaks, and soon it dies (see Figure 7.1).

Work in a number of laboratories, including our own at Rockefeller University, has shown that the pore-forming protein is part of the armamentarium of the two kinds of killer cell, the cytotoxic *T* cell

and the so-called natural killer cell. We have found a protein with a similar function in another immune cell, the eosinophil. Moreover, the same protein, or one very like it, appears to be responsible for attacks on human cells by an amoeba that causes severe dysentery.

We begin to think pore-forming proteins may be a major weapon in a wide range of cell-mediated killing. Knowing more about the process should have important medical payoffs. It may eventually be possible, for example, to treat amebic dysentery and some other parasitic, fungal and bacterial diseases by blocking a pore-forming protein. Finding a way to enhance the pore-forming process in immune-system cells might be even more important: in principle it should be helpful in the treatment of both cancer and such intractable viral diseases as AIDS.

The killer cells are elements of the cellular immune system, but their precise and lethal functioning can be studied and understood only in the context of the immune system as a whole. It has a humoral component as well as a cellular one. The humoral system defends the body primarily against bacteria and toxic molecules. Its weapons are anti-

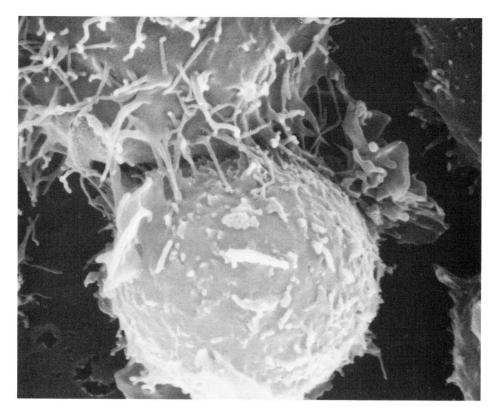

Figure 7.1 KILLER CELL is seen destroying a tumor cell. A cytotoxic *T* cell (*left, top*) makes contact with the smaller target cell. The target cell, its outer membrane shot full of holes by a protein secreted from the killer cell (*middle*), has become leaky and an influx of water has made it balloon; it has lost many of its projecting villi and there is a large

bodies, or immunoglobulins, which are synthesized and secreted by the cells called *B* lymphocytes. Each of millions of *B* cells synthesizes a particular antibody, which recognizes a particular antigen (a molecular recognition pattern); the cell displays the antibody on its surface. When the lymphocyte encounters a bacterial cell or a toxin bearing that antigen, the lymphocyte proliferates. Some of its progeny become memory cells that will respond to the same antigen faster the next time; most of the progeny become plasma cells that manufacture a large amount of the antibody and secrete it. The antibody binds to the antigen. Toxins are precipitated or otherwise neutralized by the binding itself. In the case of an invading cell the binding sets off a cascade of reactions at the cell surface involving a group of blood-serum proteins collectively known as complement. The end result of the cascade is the death of the cell.

The same precursor cells that give rise to *B* lymphocytes are the ancestors of a varied family of *T* lymphocytes that are the basis of the cellular immune system. Some *T* cells, called helper cells and suppressor cells, modulate both the humoral and the cellular system, chiefly by secreting chemical messengers called lymphokines. The major effector cell of the cellular system is the cytotoxic *T* lymphocyte, or killer *T* cell, we have mentioned. Its main targets are virus-infected cells. The other type of killer cell introduced above, the natural killer cell, is also a lymphocyte. Its precise lineage is not clear, but it seems to be closely related to the cytotoxic *T* cell. Its main targets are thought to be tumor cells, and perhaps also cells infected by agents other than viruses.

As in the case of *B* lymphocytes, the function of *T* lymphocytes depends in the first instance on proper recognition of an appropriate target. *T* cells display

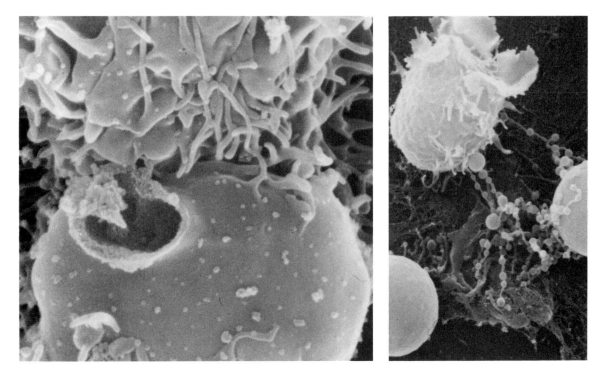

cavity in the membrane. Only the nucleus and some debris (*right*) of the target cell are left (the other nucleus is that of a second target cell). The cells were prepared by Chau-

Ching Liu and are enlarged 5,700 diameters in the first two micrographs and 4,200 diameters in the third one.

on their surface specific receptors, very similar to the B cell's antibodies, that recognize and bind to particular cell-surface antigens. T cells are more selective than B cells, however. They recognize and bind to an antigen only when it is "presented" by one of a group of surface molecules known collectively as the major histocompatibility complex (MHC). Natural killer cells, as their name implies, are less choosy about what they attack. Their receptors are less discriminating, and they are not restricted by the MHC.

Once either the killer T cell or the natural killer cell has identified its target, the killer cell binds tightly to the target cell. This close contact triggers the lethal process and also ensures that neighboring cells are not indiscriminately destroyed.

That much was known a decade ago, but the nature of the killing process continued to be a mystery. The first clues to the mystery came in the early 1970's from the laboratories of a number of investigators, notably Eric Martz of the University of Mas-

sachusetts at Amherst, Christopher S. Henney of the Immunex Corporation in Seattle, William R. Clark of the University of California at Los Angeles, Pierre Golstein of the Center for Immunology in Marseilles and Gideon Berke of the Weizmann Institute of Science in Israel. Their work dissected the killing process into a sequence of discrete stages.

First, it became clear, a "conjugate" is formed as the lymphocyte and its target come in close contact. Then some kind of lethal hit is delivered, injuring the target cell. The hit initiates what seems to be a programmed death of the injured target: death proceeds in a predetermined manner (provided only that calcium ions are present) even as the conjugate breaks up and the lymphocyte goes on to initiate a new killing cycle.

Henney and Martz were among the first to suggest that a lymphocyte appeared to kill by somehow damaging the plasma (outer) membrane of its target. Their proposal was based on their observation that radioactive molecules introduced into a target cell as markers leaked out rapidly when the target was damaged by a lymphocyte. The membrane became permeable only to markers of a certain maximum size, suggesting that the damage to the membrane might take the form of holes, or pores.

That possibility became a likelihood in 1980. Robert R. Dourmashkin and Pierre Henkart of the National Cancer Institute and their colleagues examined the surface of damaged target cells, enlarged many thousands of diameters in electron micrographs, and detected ringlike structures that appeared to be holes in the membrane. Their finding was extended three years later by Eckhard R. Podack of the New York Medical College and Gunther Dennert of the University of Southern California School of Medicine, who studied the effect of cultured killer cells on tumor cells. They established that the surface of the target cell was pocked with holes whose internal diameter ranged from five to 20 nanometers (millionths of a millimeter).

It was still not at all clear whether the pores were actually inflicted by the lymphocytes or simply reflected a terminal stage of cell death caused by some other form of injury. The search for an answer was long hampered by the lack of a ready source of killer cells. Then in 1977 Steven Gillis and Kendall A. Smith of the Dartmouth Medical School and Robert C. Gallo's group at the National Cancer Institute succeeded in maintaining mouse lymphocytes — both cytotoxic T cells and natural killer cells — in the laboratory. They were able to do so by identifying particular nutrients and growth factors required for the survival of these cells in culture; one key factor turned out to be the lymphokine called interleukin-2. Culturing made it possible to grow lymphocyte clones derived from known parent cells, and so to have at hand an abundant and homogeneous source of cytotoxic T cells and natural killer cells with known characteristics. The way was cleared for detailed analysis of such cells with the tools of cell biology and biochemistry.

An obvious feature of the lymphocytes clearly called for investigation. Micrographs had revealed numerous small, dark organelles (subcellular elements) in the cytoplasm. They appeared to be storage granules, which are common in secretory cells (see Figure 7.2). Such granules provide an efficient means of accumulating and packaging a substance synthesized by the cell so that large quantities of it can be released quickly at the right time. The release is accomplished by exocytosis: the granules move to the periphery of the cell, fuse with the plasma membrane and disgorge their contents.

Several investigators had seen that early in the cell-killing process the granules in a killer lymphocyte become concentrated in the part of the cell that is in close contact with the target. Then Abraham Kupfer and S. Jonathan Singer of the University of California at San Diego and Dennert noted that the granule-packaging Golgi apparatus seems to be directed toward that contact region and that a number of proteins of the cell's cytoskeleton (its fibrous internal framework) "reorient" toward the target cell soon after contact is established, apparently providing the motive force that redirects the Golgi and the granules.

The reorientation of the cytoskeleton and the movement of the Golgi stacks and granules take place only when and where the lymphocyte binds to an appropriate target. Roger Y. Tsien of the University of California at Berkeley showed that the binding induces an explosive increase of calcium ions in the cell; the increase triggers exocytosis. John H. Yanelli and Victor H. Engelhard of the University of Virginia have made cinemicrographs showing granules reorienting in the cytoplasm and then fusing with the plasma membrane.

All in all, the evidence suggested that contact with an appropriate target causes the killer cell to aim its secretory apparatus at the target and fire a lethal agent contained in its granules. It was necessary first to establish that the granules are in fact the shell casings and then to identify the projectile itself.

The first task was to isolate the granules and see if they alone could kill. That was done independently in 1984 by Henkart and Podack and by our group. We exploited the various techniques of subcellular fractionation, the objective of which is to break up a cell into its components and find what component contains a particular enzyme or carries out a particular function. Killer lymphocytes are broken into bits and pieces by subjecting them to pressure in nitrogen gas. The cellular debris is layered onto a density gradient of inert particles and then spun in a high-speed centrifuge. The various organelles come to rest, depending on their density, in discrete bands. We examined each of the fractions in the electron microscope and assayed them for enzymatic activity and ability to kill cells.

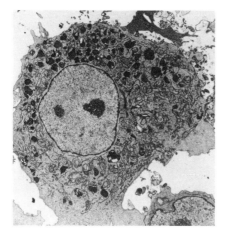 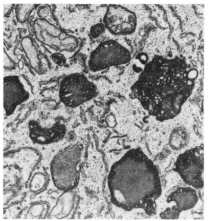

Figure 7.2 CULTURED CYTOTOXIC *T* CELL is enlarged 1,400 diameters in an electron micrograph (*left*) made by the authors with Hans Hengartner and Eckhard R. Podack. The dark storage granules in its cytoplasm, enlarged 7,600 diameters (*right*), have an electron-dense outer membrane; their amorphous matrix contains perforin, the lethal protein.

One fraction, which electron micrography showed consisted almost entirely of granules, was enriched in certain enzyme activities and was a potent killer: when the isolated granules were mixed with red blood cells or tumor cells in a medium containing calcium ions, the cells died within minutes. Electron micrographs revealed that the cells' surface carried ringlike lesions virtually indistinguishable from those produced by intact killer cells. And so the granules were shown indeed to contain the killer cells' lethal secretion.

The secreted agent itself was soon identified. In 1985, collaborating with Podack and Hans Hengartner of University Hospital in Zurich, we found a protein that all by itself (in the presence of calcium) reproduces the observed membrane lesions and the killing inflicted by intact killer cells and by granules. We isolated and purified the protein by passing extracts of granules through chromatographic columns that separated proteins on the basis of electric charge and of molecular mass, and screening the separated proteins for their efficiency in lysing red blood cells: breaking down their membrane and causing them to burst. The killer protein was isolated independently by Danielle Masson and Jürg Tschopp of the University of Lausanne.

So far only this one pore-forming protein, which is often called perforin (because it perforates membranes), has been found in the granules of cytotoxic *T* lymphocytes or natural killer cells. Its molecular mass is 70,000 daltons. Once cells are exposed to perforin in the presence of calcium ions they are lysed within a few minutes. On the other hand, if calcium ions are added to perforin before it makes contact with cells, the protein's killing activity is abolished. The effect sounds paradoxical, but actually it leads to an important insight into just how perforin kills.

The 70-kilodalton molecules secreted by a killer cell insert into the target-cell membrane. There (in the presence of calcium ions) the individual molecules (monomers) polymerize, or link up with one another. The polymer they form can assume various shapes, but under optimal conditions the final product resembles a cylinder. In the electron microscope it looks like a ring when seen in cross section and like two parallel lines when seen in longitudinal section. A fully formed ring, as Podack and Dennert first noted, ranges from five to 20 nanometers in internal diameter (see Figure 7.3).

For perforin to damage a target cell the calcium-mediated polymerization must take place entirely within the cell's membrane. The reason is that only the perforin monomer can insert into a membrane; if polymerization takes place in solution, in the absence of nearby membrane, the resultant polymer cannot enter the membrane and cannot kill. The protective effect is easy to understand. Any secreted perforin that spills into the extracellular space or the

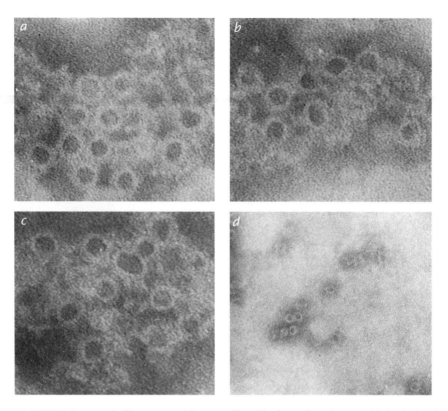

Figure 7.3 FATAL LESIONS are tubelike pores with an internal diameter of from five to 20 nanometers (millionths of a millimeter), visible in micrographs of negatively stained membrane as rings or parallel lines depending on orientation. The lesions look about the same whether in- flicted by intact lymphocytes (*a*), by isolated granules (*b*) or by perforin purified from the granules (*c*). Smaller pores (two to three nanometers in diameter) are made by a protein isolated from the amoeba *Entamoeba histolytica* (*d*).

bloodstream, where calcium is abundant, must immediately undergo polymerization and thereby be rendered inactive, virtually eliminating the possibility of "accidental" injury to nontarget cells.

On an appropriate target cell, however, the tubular pores shaped by polymerization bring about rapid, measurable changes in the target cell. The plasma membrane of a living cell retains proteins and other large molecules within the cell (except when they are to be secreted) and segregates different ions, keeping some inside and some outside the cell. The segregation of positive and negative ions establishes a transmembrane electric potential. When the membrane leaks, ions and water tend to flow down their electrochemical gradients toward equilibration, and so there is a drop in membrane potential. If the holes in the membrane are of lim-

ited size, there is an additional effect, known as the Donnan effect. The large molecules inside the membrane cannot pass through it; water and salts from the extracellular fluid pour through the membrane toward the side that has the proteins — into the cell. The cell swells, and eventually it bursts (see Figure 7.4).

By impaling target cells with microelectrodes, we were able to measure a significant drop in membrane potential soon after perforin was administered. With sensitive electronic equipment we were even able to measure the ion current flowing through individual pores. Our results were consistent with the predictions of the Donnan effect. The measurements showed, moreover, that the perforin holes are stable structures that persist as open pathways in the membrane. By determining just which

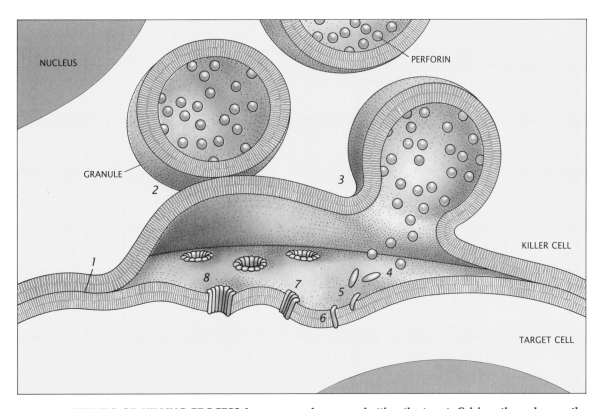

Figure 7.4 DETAILS OF KILLING PROCESS have now been elucidated. A rise in the lymphocyte's calcium-ion level, apparently triggered by the receptor-mediated binding of the killer cell to its target (*1*), brings about exocytosis, in which the granules fuse with the cell membrane (*2*) and disgorge their perforin (*3*) into the small intercellular space abutting the target. Calcium there changes the conformation of the individual perforin molecules, or monomers (*4*), which then bind to the target-cell membrane (*5*) and insert into it (*6*). The monomers polymerize like staves of a barrel (*7*) to form pores (*8*) that admit water and salts and kill the cell.

ions and small molecules got through the damaged membrane, we were able to estimate that the functional internal diameter of the pores ranges from one to 10 nanometers (as opposed to the observed diameter in micrographs of from five to 20 nanometers).

Given the apparently undiscriminating efficiency of perforin as a killer, how can one account for the specificity of killing by lymphocytes? We have mentioned that "accidental" killing by perforin that gets away from the lymphocyte-target interface is prevented by calcium-induced polymerization of the protein. What one might term "purposeful" killing of nontarget cells (as a result of contact with a killer lymphocyte) is prevented, on the other hand, by the lymphocyte's ability to rec-

ognize an appropriate cell—one displaying, for example, either viral antigens or tumor antigens. In other words, the specificity of killing resides solely in the requirement for close contact, which depends in turn on the binding of killer cell to target cell through the interaction of antigens on the target cell with receptors on the killer cell.

But what keeps the killer cell from killing itself? It cannot be the close-contact requirement, since the killer cell's membrane is continually exposed directly to a secreted perforin. Chau-Ching Liu, a graduate student in our laboratory, and one of us (Young) collaborated with Clark recently to show that even purified perforin fails to kill either cytotoxic *T* cells or natural killer cells. The self-protective mechanism is not known, but we have a hypothesis. We think the killer-cell membrane may incorporate a special protein, which we call protectin, that is very similar to perforin (see Figure 7.5). The close homology would promote a kind of "faulty polymerization": the protectin would rapidly combine with any perforin monomer that gets to the killer-cell membrane, thereby preventing either the insertion of perforin into the membrane or the normal perforin-to-perforin polymerization that would form a pore. We are now engaged in an intensive search for our hypothetical protein.

All the recent studies we have described here were done with mouse-lymphocyte cultures maintained in the laboratory. It was conceivable that perforin was just a laboratory curiosity and not truly the lymphocytes' weapon in vivo. Collaborating with Bice Perussia of the Wistar Institute in Philadelphia and Liu, we looked for perforin in lymphocytes freshly obtained from human blood. We could find none. When the lymphocytes were stimulated

with interleukin-2, however, they proliferated in vitro and began to synthesize perforin. We found this to be the case for both cytotoxic T cells and natural killer cells; similar results have been reported by Leora S. Zalman and Hans J. Muller-Eberhard of the Research Institute of Scripps Clinic and their colleagues. The in vitro effect of interleukin-2 presumably reflects its effect in the body, where it is produced by helper T cells and promotes a range of immune responses.

Indeed, the effect we noted in the laboratory may explain an apparent clinical effect of interleukin-2 first reported in 1984 by Steven A. Rosenberg of the National Cancer Institute. He devised a novel therapy for certain intractable cancers in which lymphocytes extracted from the blood of a patient are stimulated with interleukin-2 outside the body and then infused back into the patient. The lymphocytes are presumably thereby activated to kill more effi-

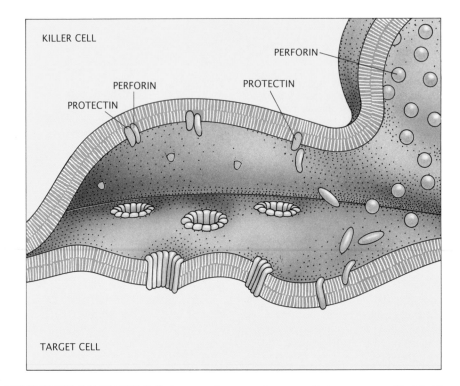

Figure 7.5 PROTECTIVE MECHANISM that prevents self-inflicted death of the killer cell has been postulated by the authors. They think a protein, protectin, that is very similar to perforin is concentrated in the lymphocyte membrane; perforin monomers bind to the protectin and are prevented from polymerizing to form pores in the killer-cell membrane.

ciently; some tumor regression has been observed in some patients. The procedure is highly toxic and therefore still in an experimental stage, but a better understanding of how to induce the expression of perforin by killer lymphocytes will certainly have a role in designing immunotherapies for cancer.

Although it seems clear that killer cells kill by punching holes in target-cell membranes, the lymphocytes may have other weapons too. John H. Russell of Washington University in St. Louis has put forward an "internal disintegration" model to explain the killing event. The model is based on the observation that early in the course of target-cell injury the membrane enclosing the nucleus of the cell ruptures and the DNA in the nucleus breaks up into small fragments. Russell and others argue that the death of the target cell results from the cleaving of the DNA, which is presumably triggered by some signal emitted by the killer cell. The model has not been elaborated in detail, but it cannot be excluded by our findings. Perhaps there are several different killing mechanisms.

Indeed, we have found that certain cytotoxic T-cell lines maintained in culture for some time continue to exert killing activity even though they do not secrete perforin. Do they secrete something else? We have preliminary evidence that a molecule we call leukalexin, which kills cells over the course of several hours rather than minutes, may be present in killer cells. It is just possible that even if perforin pores first admit only water and salts and are too small to pass most proteins, they eventually enlarge enough (through additional polymerization) to admit one chain of a protein—perhaps leukalexin—that cleaves DNA. Alternatively, pore formation might lead eventually to the admission of a DNA-cleaving protein by somehow promoting endocytosis, the process by which large molecules are generally taken into cells.

Pore formation may not be the only killing mechanism for killer lymphocytes, but it is clearly an efficient one. It figures, for example, in humoral immunity as well as in cellular immunity: it is the end result of the complement cascade that kills bacteria labeled by antibodies (see Figure 7.6). The terminal proteins of the cascade polymerize to form holes, much like the pores made of perforin, with an internal diameter of 10 nanometers. Podack and we have found, as has Tschopp independently, that the

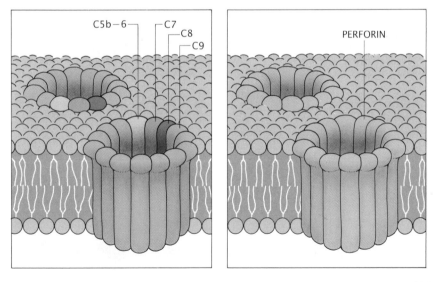

Figure 7.6 HUMORAL IMMUNE SYSTEM forms pores much like those inflicted by the cellular system's killer lymphocytes. Binding of antibodies to a target cell triggers a cascade in which successive proteins of the complement system are activated. Eventually the protein C5b-6 binds to the target's surface membrane, after which C7, C8 and a number of C9 proteins aggregate to form a pore (*left*). In contrast, the pores made by killer cells are formed by the self-aggregation of one kind of subunit: the perforin monomer (*right*).

terminal complement proteins have significant homology with perforin: the sequence of amino acids (the building blocks of proteins) is identical in some parts of these complement proteins and of perforin. This similarity between elements of the humoral and the cellular immune systems cannot have come about by accident. We speculate that the killer proteins of both systems had a common ancestry but diverged somewhat to become specialized for their respective roles. Once an efficient mechanism evolves in an organism, it tends to be well conserved by natural selection.

Cell killing is not limited to immune cells, or indeed to organisms of higher complexity. Numerous species, including certain bacteria, fungi and protozoan parasites, are effective killers of cells. Among the weapons many of them have in common are proteins that punch holes in the surface of a target cell. We chose to study one such species in an attempt to improve our understanding of how lymphocytes kill their targets. Certain virulent strains of the amoeba *Entamoeba histolytica* infect human beings worldwide, invading the intestine to cause severe dysentery and often spreading to other organs. In a laboratory culture these strains kill a wide range of cells, in each case first binding tightly to the target (see Figure 7.7).

In 1982 Carlos Gitler of the Weizmann Institute and we independently isolated from *E. histolytica* a protein that forms pores in the surface membrane of target cells. The purified pore-forming protein is a potent killer. This PFP, as we first named it, is much smaller than perforin (14,000 daltons), but like perforin it polymerizes and forms large tubular lesions,

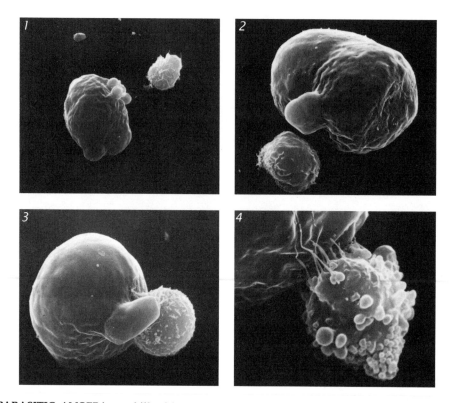

Figure 7.7 PARASITIC AMOEBA can kill with a pore-forming protein that has the same effect as perforin. In these micrographs (*Entamoeba histolytica* (the larger cell) approaches its target, an immune-system macrophage (*1*), and extends a pseudopod (*2*). After making contact the amoeba may kill its target by phagocytosis, or ingestion (*3*), or instead may secrete its lethal pore-forming protein, which causes the target to swell and show extensive blebbing, or blistering (*4*), and then to die.

with an internal diameter of from two to three nanometers, in a cell membrane. We think the amoeba kills by binding to its target and shooting it full of holes made of a PFP polymer. The similarity of the killing mechanisms in killer cells that attack the body and killer cells that defend it would seem to be a nice example of convergence in evolution. The amoeba and the human lymphocytes have independently developed functionally similar pore-forming proteins that accomplish the same objective: the death of cells.

AUTOIMMUNITY AND CELLULAR THERAPY

· · ·

Introduction

The immune response has enormous clinical relevance in its role as a protection against infectious agents. However, the potent effector mechanisms that the immune system can marshall against foreign antigens can be devastating if they are turned against self antigens. Unfortunately, such a misguided response may occur with sufficient frequency that autoimmune diseases are clinical problems of considerable magnitude. Among the most important disorders in which immune responses lead to severe damage of self tissues are systemic lupus erythematosus, rheumatoid arthritis, insulin-dependent diabetes mellitus and, very likely, multiple sclerosis.

The mechanisms that underlie these disorders are not well understood; it is not clear why immune responses against self-antigens develop in individuals with these diseases. It still remains to be established whether these autoimmune responses represent a failure of the natural induction of tolerance or whether they are induced as the result of an unusual type of infectious process that leads to the activation of T cell clones that are not normally activated.

Chapter 8, "The Self, the World and Autoimmunity," by Irun R. Cohen, deals with the problems of autoimmunity and autoimmune diseases in general and then treats the problem of an experimental autoimmune arthritis of mice in greater detail. The various mechanisms that can underlie the deranged responses in these diseases are considered and a novel form of therapy, based on the induction of an immune response specific for the T cells that mediate autoimmunity is discussed. The concept of the autoaggressive T cell used as a "vaccine" (i.e., a "T Cell vaccine") to induce a response that somehow eliminates or neutralizes autoaggression is an exciting one. Continued work in this area will be essential to obtain a picture of the general applicability of this approach to dealing with autoimmune responses.

The growth of knowledge about the functions of lymphokines has raised the possibility that these molecules could be used therapeutically. GM-CSF and IL-3 have promise as agents to regulate the levels of white blood cells in patients with depressed bone marrow function, most particularly in individuals who are being aggressively treated with chemotherapeutic drugs for cancer. IFNγ has been the subject of intense interest as an anti-cancer drug. One of the other interferons, IFNα, has proven to be very effective in the treatment of hairy cell leukemia.

The alternative of neutralizing the function of lymphokines and related molecules has considerable potential. Molecules such as IL-1, IL-6 and TNF play important roles in inflammatory diseases, and approaches to inhibit their function under controlled conditions might be of value in limiting tissue damage in inflammation. In rodents IL-4 is central to the production of antibodies that cause allergic responses (antibodies of the IgE class). Neutralizing IL-4 prevents IgE responses suggesting that blocking the action or production of IL-4 in humans might be very useful in the prevention or treatment of allergies. The recent demonstration that receptors for several of the lymphokines are made in a soluble form as well as in the form of membrane-bound molecules raises the possibility that these natural, soluble lymphokine-binding molecules could be safely used as inhibiters of lymphokine function.

Chapter 9, "Adoptive Immunotherapy for Cancer," by Steven Rosenberg, describes an ambitious combination of the use of lymphokines and lymphocytes. Rosenberg and his colleagues at the National Cancer Institute have pioneered the idea that the antitumor action of autologous lymphocytes of the individual could be used therapeutically. Their approach is to expand the patient's cells in vitro and to return them to the patient together with lymphokines that would sustain their growth and function in vivo. Thus far, two major types of such adoptive therapy have been examined. One is based on a set of lymphoid cells that have a potent but nonspecific antitumor activity. These cells have been designated lymphokine-activated killer (LAK) cells and appear to be related to natural killer (NK) cells. The cells can be obtained from the patients, expanded in vitro with IL-2 and then returned to the patient with large amounts of IL-2. This therapy has had some promising results. Nonetheless, the use of large amounts of IL-2 is not without considerable toxicity. More recently, antigen-specific killer cells found infiltrating tumors (tumor-infiltrating lymphocytes) have been used in a strategy analogous to that developed for LAK cells. The cells are expanded in vitro with IL-2 and then returned to the patient, who receives large amounts of IL-2 to sustain their proliferation and activity.

Rosenberg and his colleagues hope to expand the potential of this approach by introducing genes into tumor-infiltrating lymphocytes that could endow them with superior antitumor activity, thus combining the natural activity of the cells with functions based on the products of genes, such as that for tumor necrosis factor.

The Self, the World and Autoimmunity

Autoimmunity—in which the immune system recognizes and attacks the self's own tissues—is not as simple as it seemed. Self-recognition appears to be at the heart of health as well as of certain diseases.

. . .

Irun R. Cohen
April, 1988

It is generally assumed that the main job of the immune system is to distinguish between what is "self" and what is "not self." Once the distinction has been made, "self" is preserved and "not self" is destroyed. At the most general level, of course, this is true, and human beings remain alive and healthy only because it is so. Recently it has become clear, however, that at a finer level of detail the distinction between self and other is not absolute. One of the paths to this insight has been provided by the autoimmune disorders, in which the immune system attacks normal, healthy tissue. Autoimmune disease, which may be crippling or fatal, can strike any tissue or organ. Its victims are often in the prime of life, and for unknown reasons they are more frequently women than men.

Work in my laboratory on a form of autoimmune arthritis shows that the basis of autoimmunity may be a resemblance between a specific foreign molecule and a molecule of the self. What is more, our work is consistent with a model of the immune system in which the immune-system receptors that perform the work of recognition can themselves be recognized by other receptors. Such "self-recognition," which was strictly outlawed by older models of the immune system, may form the basis of a

network whose equilibrium keeps the body healthy. When it is disrupted, as it is in autoimmunity, disease results. This new picture, in which self and world are no longer absolutely distinct, has already begun to yield practical benefit in the form of vaccines that may ultimately ease the substantial suffering caused by autoimmune diseases.

The list of autoimmune diseases is both long and disturbing. It includes multiple sclerosis, in which the tissue attacked is myelin (a substance that sheaths nerves in the central nervous system); myasthenia gravis, in which the target is a receptor molecule for the important neurotransmitter acetylcholine; rheumatoid arthritis, whose target is the peripheral joints; type I (juvenile) diabetes mellitus, in which the cells producing insulin are destroyed, and systemic lupus erythematosis, in which DNA, blood vessels, skin and kidneys are attacked. In contrast to AIDS, which is marked by an inactivation of key cells in the immune system, in all these diseases the immunological response is strong and well-focused; it is, however, directed at some essential component of the body. The immune system is itself the culprit. How can that be?

Clearly the answer lies in the problem of recognition. That problem in turn touches on the cells that mediate recognition in the immune system: the lymphocytes. The immune system includes two such classes of cells, which are called T lymphocytes and B lymphocytes. Both types arise from stem cells in the bone marrow. The stem cells, however, lack the receptors that enable B and T cells to recognize specific molecules as targets for immune attack. Such immune receptors appear as the multipotential stem cells mature. As a result of the process of maturation, each B or T cell ultimately comes to have many copies of one immune receptor on its surface and therefore is able to recognize only one other molecule. Any molecule so recognized is called an antigen.

One of the remarkable features of the process of recognition is that it requires not the whole antigen but only a small piece known as an epitope. If (as is often the case) the molecule to be recognized is a polymer such as a protein or a sugar chain, the epitope frequently consists of as a few as from four to six of its thousands of monomeric subunits (amino acids in proteins, sugar units in sugar chains). The shape and the electric charge of each epitope are such that it will best fit a particular receptor. When an epitope finds its complementary receptor, they form a reversible association that generates a signal in the T or B cell.

At the heart of this process is the fact that each lymphocyte bears receptors with but a single specificity. For the immune system to be able to recognize a wide range of pathogens, however, there must be a great diversity of receptors, and indeed new receptors are constantly being produced at random by a process of genetic recombination in the progenitor stem cells. Not all the receptors created in this way are equally useful, and the immune system weeds out the unnecessary ones by a process called clonal selection. The lymphocyte whose receptor happens to have the closest fit to an epitope on a microbial antigen enjoys an advantage over its competitors: it replicates faster, and soon it may come to predominate over the other T and B cells in its vicinity.

The descendants of the progenitor make up a clone that not only increases in size but also differentiates into specialized forms. B cells may become plasma cells, which secrete antibodies (molecules with the same shape as the clone's antigen receptor), or memory cells, which persist to identify the epitope with increased efficiency if the pathogen returns. T cells mature into one group bearing a surface marker known as T4 and another bearing a marker known as T8. Within each group are cells that act directly ("effectors") and others that act by influencing other immune-system cells ("regulators"). T8 effectors are cytotoxic: they kill cells bearing a specific antigen. T8 regulators are suppressive: they inhibit the activities of other T or B cells. T4 effectors damage tissue by activating other white cells; T4 regulatory cells are "helpers" that facilitate the action of both B and T cells.

Now, the random generation of new receptors and their winnowing by clonal selection endows the immune system with great flexibility. The number of possible receptor structures is enormous: perhaps millions of different T-lymphocyte clones and hundreds of millions of B-lymphocyte clones. From the randomly generated receptors that are continually being produced, clonal selection narrows the field to a few dominant types for each antigen. From a theoretical point of view clonal selection can be seen as a form of digital processing, in which the system is able to direct its attention to the most relevant information (the receptor that best fits an epitope) and disregard the rest (all, or almost all, competing receptor-epitope pairs).

Yet that very flexibility is the source of a problem: self-recognition. If the immune system can recognize almost anything, why not the molecules that belong to the self? F. Macfarlane Burnet of the University of Melbourne, author of the theory of clonal selection, proposed a solution to the problem of self-recognition. During prenatal development, Burnet argued, all the antigens that were present would be self antigens. If recognition of an epitope during gestation triggered clonal suicide, the immune system would be purged of all self-recognized clones (see Figure 8.1). Recognition of epitopes after birth would induce active immunity, but by then the immune system would be blind to self structures. Burnet explained the appearance of autoimmune disease by exposure after birth to self-antigens that had been accidentally sequestered during gestation.

To be reliable, however, clonal elimination requires distinguishing absolutely between self and not-self: receptors that recognize self must be eliminated and those that do not must be spared. Yet it seems clear that such an absolute distinction cannot easily be made. One reason is that although the receptor-antigen relation is generally thought of as a lock-and-key affair, in reality the fit is not exact or exclusive. Within certain limits a single receptor can combine with many different epitopes, each of

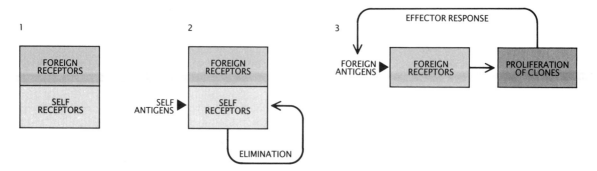

Figure 8.1 CLONAL SUICIDE was a theory developed to account for the absence of autoimmune disease in most people. A clone is a group of cells descended from the same progenitor and hence genetically identical. The immune system can create clones capable of recognizing both self and foreign antigens (1). In clonal suicide all clones having receptors for self antigens are eliminated before birth (2). Clones that recognize foreign antigens persist. On encountering the corresponding antigen, they proliferate and differentiate to combat the invader (3). It has become clear that self and foreign antigens cannot be distinguished by such a simple mechanism.

which it fits with greater or lesser precision. The capacity of millions of different receptors to bind many epitopes enlarges the functional repertoire so greatly that it is difficult to imagine that any biological molecule could pass unrecognized by at least one receptor—including the molecules of the self.

The challenge is compounded by the fact that the self and the invader are made up of the same building blocks: proteins, carbohydrates, nucleic acids and lipids. What is more, molecules such as enzymes or hormones that perform key biological functions tend to be conserved in evolution so that self and invader may have identical—or at least very similar—molecules. Finally, it seems that some pathogens actually make hostlike antigens as a means of disguise. For example, leishmania parasites synthesize antigens similar to those of the red blood cells of their mammalian hosts. It appears that antigenic "mimicry" is a persistent feature of the struggle between self and pathogen.

To understand the role of antigenic mimicry in autoimmunity my colleagues and I studied an experimental disease of rats called adjuvant arthritis, which was first observed by Carl M. Pearson of the University of California at Los Angeles in the 1950's. Pearson noted that rats inoculated with a mixture of mineral oil and killed organisms of *Mycobacterium tuberculosis* (the tuberculosis agent) developed arthritis (see Figure 8.2). Adjuvant arthritis caused degeneration of the cartilage in the joints, and its symptoms, Pearson and others noted, were much like those of rheumatoid arthritis. Rheuma-

toid arthritis is typically manifested as a progressive inflammation of hands and feet. Unlike osteoarthritis (which often accompanies aging), rheumatoid arthritis typically strikes young women, and it can lead to tragic deformity.

Since both rheumatoid and adjuvant arthritis were assumed to be due to autoimmunity, my co-workers and I hoped that explication of the disorder in rats would help us to understand the human disease. The tissue damage seen in adjuvant arthritis was characteristic of T lymphocytes rather than B lymphocytes or other immune components, and so our strategy was to isolate the clones of T cells that were attacking the cartilage in the rats' joints. Although the strategy sounds simple, in actuality it required some substantial technical advances, most of which were due to the pioneering work of Avraham Ben-Nun, who was then one of my graduate students.

Ben-Nun's work was based on another induced autoimmune disorder, known as experimental autoimmune encephalomyelitis (EAE). Considerably more was known about EAE than about adjuvant arthritis. It could be induced in laboratory animals by inoculation with basic protein, a component of myelin in the central nervous system. The immunity to basic protein is manifested by paralysis (often fatal) and inflammation in the region of the brain and spinal cord where the nerve fibers are sheathed in myelin. Some workers consider EAE to be the best laboratory model of multiple sclerosis, and much

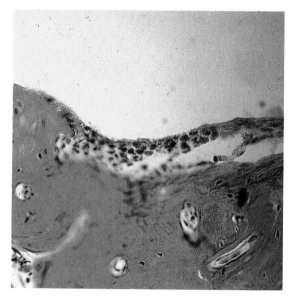
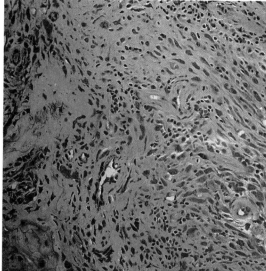

Figure 8.2 CARTILAGE DAMAGE, hallmark of adjuvant arthritis, results when *T* lymphocytes attack joint cartilage. The micrograph at the left shows rat joint tissue eight days after inoculation with an "adjuvant" containing ground-up *Mycobacterium tuberculosis* (the tuberculosis pathogen) in mineral oil. Lymphocytes have begun to invade the cartilage (*upper layer of tissue*). The micrograph at the right, made 27 days later, shows the normal cartilage architecture extensively disrupted by white blood cells.

work had gone toward characterizing the epitopes of basic protein that are responsible for EAE in rats, guinea pigs and mice as well as in other experimental animals.

Like adjuvant arthritis, EAE was thought to be caused by *T* cells rather than *B* cells or antibodies, and our strategy was to isolate clones of *T* cells that responded specifically to basic protein. Ben-Nun worked out a method for growing such clones. *T* cells from rats immunized against basic protein were grown in a culture medium containing the basic-protein antigen. Although the cells that recognized basic protein were a small minority, the presence of their antigen stimulated them to proliferate at the expense of the other lymphocytes: it was clonal selection in tissue culture. That procedure enabled us (in this work Ben-Nun and I collaborated with Hartmut Wekerle, then at the Max Planck Institute for Immunobiology in West Germany) to obtain pure clones of *T* cells that respond to basic protein; all the clones isolated so far have been of the *T*4 type.

Further work showed unequivocally that these *T*4 cells cause EAE. Yaakov Naparstek showed that they accumulate in the brain and spinal cord just before the onset of paralysis. Moreover, we were able to retrieve anti-basic-protein *T* cells from immunized rats and, by injecting them, cause EAE in other rats. This was the first time a specific clone of *T* cells had been shown without question to be responsible for a known autoimmune disorder. Paradoxically, although the *T* cells from the immunized rats were able to cause disease, in some instances the rats they were taken from had already recovered from their severe paralysis and seemed to be clinically well. That perplexing finding implied the existence of mechanisms for holding autoimmunity in check—a subject to which I shall return.

Soon after these experiments were done, Joseph Holoshitz, who was spending a leave in my laboratory, suggested that we apply our experience with EAE to adjuvant arthritis. It seemed a sound idea. The catch was that in the case of EAE the antigen that caused the disorder—basic protein—was well known to begin with. In the case of adjuvant arthritis, however, the relevant antigen was not known. It was assumed that the antigen must be one belonging to *Mycobacterium tuberculosis*, but *M. tubercu-*

losis includes many thousands of antigens. How could we find the antigenic needle in this immunologic stack?

We reasoned that only the human investigators on the case were ignorant of the right antigen. Surely the *T* lymphocytes that cause the disorder recognize the relevant antigen. Accordingly, Holoshitz cultured cells from arthritic rats with pulverized *M. tuberculosis* organisms. If antigenic mimicry was indeed at work and there existed bacterial antigens resembling the self antigens that were under attack in the arthritic rats, the disease-causing *T* cells might pick them out from among all the other bacterial antigens. When that happened, the relevant clone would predominate by clonal selection. That is just what happened. The second *T*-lymphocyte line that was obtained was found to induce arthritis when injected into rats. Holoshitz went on to isolate a clone called A2b that caused even more severe disease.

Having induced the bacterial antigen to pick out the relevant *T*-cell clone, we could now employ the *T* cells to find the antigen itself. That work was undertaken by Willem van Eden, who came to my laboratory as a postdoctoral fellow from the Netherlands. Van Eden cultured clone A2b with fractions of ground-up *M. tuberculosis* organisms and with various components of joint tissue. As expected, A2b recognized a mycobacterial fraction (one prepared by my colleague Ayalla Frenkel). In addition the clone recognized proteoglycan, a joint-cartilage molecule that includes sugar and protein components (see Figure 8.3). As it happens, the epitope recognized by A2b was on the part of the proteoglycan molecule called the core protein.

This double recognition was exciting, because it amounted to antigenic mimicry in the test tube: a clone of *T* cells with a single specificity had recognized both a foreign antigen and a self antigen. Adjuvant arthritis could now be explained as the result of a resemblance between those antigens.

But what were the precise epitopes involved? Van Eden's initial work had identified only a fraction of ground-up bacterium, not a specific epitope. To identify a specific epitope we needed to separate *M. tuberculosis* organisms into their component molecules and determine which molecule was recognized by A2b. Once the molecule had been identified we could break it down into progressively smaller pieces until we found the smallest defined

piece A2b would recognize, which would constitute the relevant epitope.

Although the process is simple to describe, it might not have been possible without a useful trick of genetic engineering. Mycobacteria are notoriously difficult to study biochemically. Hence biochemists have resorted to inserting their genes into *Escherichia coli*, a well-behaved and much studied laboratory pet. When the genes are expressed by *E. coli*, large amounts of mycobacterial antigens are made available for study. The availability of such "expression libraries" of *M. tuberculosis* proteins offered us a relatively simple way of identifying the antigens that had been recognized by clone A2b.

Van Eden tested the responses of A2b to an expression library prepared by Jan D. A. van Embden and Jelle E. R. Thole of the National Institute of Public Health and Environmental Hygiene in the Netherlands. To our delight A2b responded to one of the mycobacterial gene products, a protein with a molecular weight of about 65,000, the amino acid sequence of which had already been worked out. Thole and Embden obtained fragments of the protein and tested them against A2b. Ruurd van der Zee of the State University of Groningen then synthesized amino acid chains spanning the area of the protein likely to contain the relevant epitope. The chains were tested and the epitope, consisting of nine amino acids, was identified.

The precise resemblance between the bacterial epitope and the protein part of the proteoglycan remains to be specified. Fortunately the amino acid sequences of proteoglycans have been worked out quite thoroughly. The nine amino acids of the bacterial epitope were compared with published core-protein sequences, and a resemblance was found to a stretch of the link protein that joins the core protein to the proteoglycan's sugar backbone. Four of the nine amino acids in the two stretches are identical. We are currently testing whether that resemblance could account for the double recognition of the two epitopes by clone A2b and therefore for the autoimmunity that underlies adjuvant arthritis.

Does such molecular mimicry also have a role in causing rheumatoid arthritis in human beings? Although there is no definitive answer, early findings are suggestive. We investigated immune responses of some 50 patients suffering from rheumatoid arthritis or from a nonautoimmune degenerative dis-

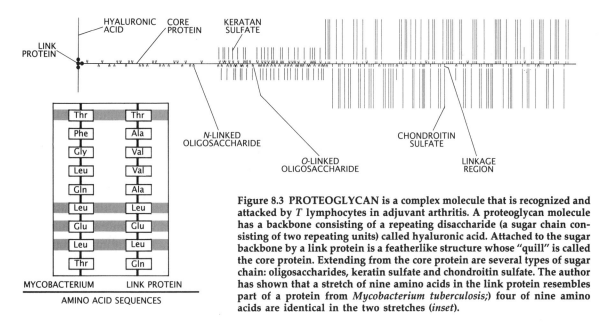

Figure 8.3 PROTEOGLYCAN is a complex molecule that is recognized and attacked by *T* lymphocytes in adjuvant arthritis. A proteoglycan molecule has a backbone consisting of a repeating disaccharide (a sugar chain consisting of two repeating units) called hyaluronic acid. Attached to the sugar backbone by a link protein is a featherlike structure whose "quill" is called the core protein. Extending from the core protein are several types of sugar chain: oligosaccharides, keratin sulfate and chondroitin sulfate. The author has shown that a stretch of nine amino acids in the link protein resembles part of a protein from *Mycobacterium tuberculosis;*) four of nine amino acids are identical in the two stretches (*inset*).

ease of the joints. *T* lymphocytes from both groups were exposed to a mycobacterial fraction containing the cartilage-mimicking epitope. The cells from the rheumatoid arthritis patients underwent a markedly augmented proliferation; those from the others showed a much lower rate of proliferation that was comparable to the rate in healthy people.

Rheumatoid arthritis does appear to be associated with a specific reactivity of *T* cells to a mycobacterial antigen. Such findings, however, by no means establish a causal relationship. The reactivity of the *T* lymphocytes might be the result of arthritis rather than its cause. For example, rheumatoid arthritis might trigger a response of *T* cells to cartilage proteoglycans. The *T* cells might then cross-react to mycobacterial epitopes that happen to resemble the cartilage antigens. There is certainly no obvious connection between *M. tuberculosis* infection and the subsequent development of rheumatoid arthritis. Yet nonvirulent mycobacteria are ubiquitous, and perhaps a clinically invisible exposure might later lead to autoimmunity.

Such connections are known for other pathogens. Acute rheumatic fever, for example, a condition characterized by inflammation of the heart, joints and nervous system, is almost always preceded by an acute infection (usually of the throat and tonsils) with a type of streptococcal bacterium. In the 1960's

Melvin H. Kaplan of Case Western Reserve University showed that antibodies made by rabbits against streptococcal antigens also bind to human heart tissue. It should be noted, however, that although all the streptococci of a particular strain may carry human-mimicking epitopes, only a small minority of infected people ever come down with acute rheumatic fever. Moreover, the autoimmune attack is generally brief. It would seem that the immune system has the capacity to regulate autoimmunity. How?

Surprisingly, the great scope of the receptor repertoire, which causes the problem by encompassing both the self and the world, may also provide a solution. In the early 1970's Niels Kaj Jerne of the Basel Institute for Immunology formulated a theory of immunity based on observations by several investigators that antigen receptors could themselves be recognized by other receptors on lymphocytes or antibodies. A receptor could also be an antigen! Therefore in addition to receptors for each epitope (as postulated by Burnet), Jerne's conception included receptors for each receptor [see "The Immune System," by Niels Kaj Jerne; SCIENTIFIC AMERICAN, July, 1973]. The original Burnetian specificity of the receptor is referred to as its idiotype, and the specificity of the receptor's receptor is called the anti-idiotype.

That concept has some remarkable implications. If the epitope is thought of as a key and the idiotypic receptor as a lock, what of the anti-idiotypic receptor? Because it is complementary to the idiotype (the lock), the anti-idiotypic receptor must have the form of the key (see Figure 8.4). The key, however, is also the form of the epitope. Hence the epitope and the anti-idiotypic receptor may have the same shape. Jerne argued that in addition to a set of receptors complementary to the antigenic world, the immune system contains a set of receptors (the anti-idiotypic ones) that are homologous to the antigenic world: the system contains not only itself but also the world. This self-recognizing network establishes an equilibrium that regulates the behavior of the immune system, according to Jerne.

Jerne's ideas have generated many experiments, and results are accumulating that support the network concept. Several workers have found that immunization with an epitope leads to the production of antibodies complementary to the epitope, followed thereafter by the production of anti-idiotypic antibodies that mimic the shape of the epitope. Yoram Shechter, Ruth Maron, Dana Elias and I carried out such experiments in mice (see Figure 8.5). We employed an insulin epitope and obtained an anti-idiotypic antibody that resembles the relevant part of the insulin molecule. (In fact, we are now finding anti-idiotypic, insulin-mimicking antibodies in the blood of some people suffering from the autoimmune form of diabetes. What these antibodies are doing there is still a mystery.) On a more practical level, it is hoped that anti-idiotypic antibodies can be exploited for vaccines: the anti-idiotype mimics the shape of a microbial epitope (and so induces immunity) but is harmless.

If recognition of self through the formation of anti-idiotypic receptors is central to the immune system, what distinguishes between healthy self-recognition and autoimmune disease? Immunologists who accept Jerne's ideas would propose that an equilibrium between idiotypic and anti-idiotypic receptors somehow yields a tolerance to self-epi-

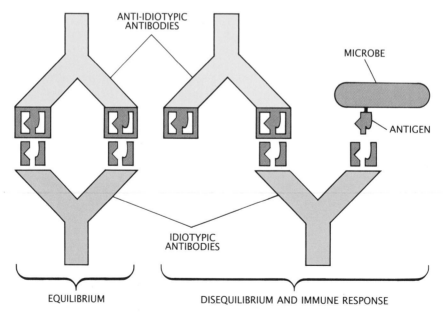

Figure 8.4 ANTI-IDIOTYPE NETWORK may underlie the immune system's response to disease. The idiotype is a receptor's specificity for an antigen. The anti-idiotype is a second receptor's lock-and-key fit with the first. Under ordinary, equilibrium conditions, idiotypic anti-idiotypic receptors may bind, holding each other in check (*left*). If a microbial antigen is present, it binds to an idiotypic receptor, creating a disequilibrium that leads to the immune response (*right*). It is also possible that the equilibrium between idiotypes and anti-idiotypes somehow restrains the harmful effects of autoimmunity.

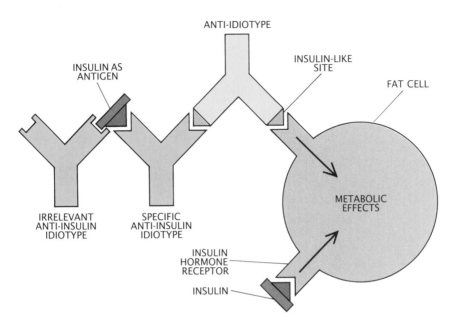

ANTI-IDIOTYPE

INSULIN AS ANTIGEN

INSULIN-LIKE SITE

FAT CELL

IRRELEVANT ANTI-INSULIN IDIOTYPE

SPECIFIC ANTI-INSULIN IDIOTYPE

METABOLIC EFFECTS

INSULIN HORMONE RECEPTOR

INSULIN

Figure 8.5 HORMONES CAN BE SHORT-CIRCUITED by the effects of the idiotype–anti-idiotype network, as is shown in a schematic representation of work done in the author's laboratory. Mice immunized to the hormone insulin develop antibodies to several structures on the insulin molecule, including the part (*red*) that binds to the insulin receptor of fat cells. The mice then spontaneously develop anti-idiotypic antibodies that bind to the idiotypic receptor. The receptors of the anti-idiotypic antibodies resemble the configuration of the part of insulin that binds to the insulin receptor. Hence the anti-idiotypic receptors also bind to the insulin receptor, eliciting metabolic effects normally caused by insulin.

topes and prevents autoimmune disease. Harmful self-recognition, they would argue, is checked by the mesh of the network and not merely by the presence or absence of a specific antigen. Indeed, it does seem that the immune system can live with and control autoimmunity. As I mentioned above, T lymphocytes capable of causing EAE can persist in rats that have recovered from the disease, and people do recover from rheumatic fever and other autoimmune disorders.

Although the network model offers a convincing interpretation of autoimmunity, it has not been conclusively established. Even without full theoretical understanding, however, the first practical steps have been taken toward preventing and treating autoimmune diseases. Having in hand the specific T lymphocyte clones responsible for EAE, adjuvant arthritis and some other experimental diseases, we decided to find out whether they could be used as "vaccines" against autoimmunity.

The first step was to take the line of anti-basic-protein T cells responsible for EAE and subject them to gamma radiation. The treated cells lost their virulence and were no longer able to induce EAE when they were injected into rats. The animals into which the T cells were injected, however, acquired permanent resistance to EAE: immunization of the rats with basic protein no longer triggered an attack on tissues of the central nervous system. The rats were perfectly capable of responding to other antigens and could even develop adjuvant arthritis when they were exposed to *M. tuberculosis* antigens. We had achieved an experimental vaccine. Its basis was immunizing the rats against the T cells, which had receptors for basic protein.

Vaccination with T lymphocytes was quickly extended to adjuvant arthritis (see Figure 8.6). In collaboration with my colleague Meir Sinitzky we found that the potency of the "vaccine" could be considerably enhanced by aggregating the receptors

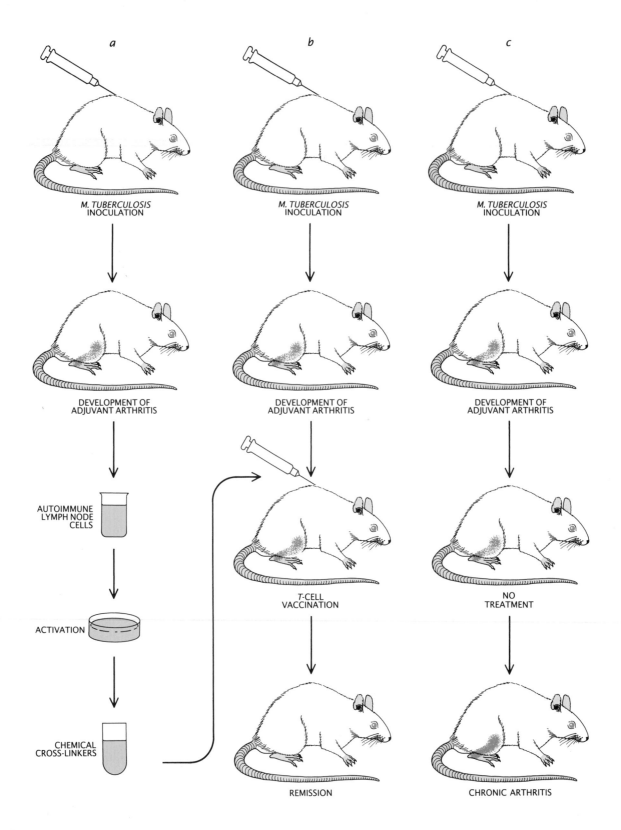

a

b

c

M. TUBERCULOSIS
INOCULATION

M. TUBERCULOSIS
INOCULATION

M. TUBERCULOSIS
INOCULATION

DEVELOPMENT OF
ADJUVANT ARTHRITIS

DEVELOPMENT OF
ADJUVANT ARTHRITIS

DEVELOPMENT OF
ADJUVANT ARTHRITIS

AUTOIMMUNE
LYMPH NODE
CELLS

ACTIVATION

CHEMICAL
CROSS-LINKERS

T-CELL
VACCINATION

NO
TREATMENT

REMISSION

CHRONIC ARTHRITIS

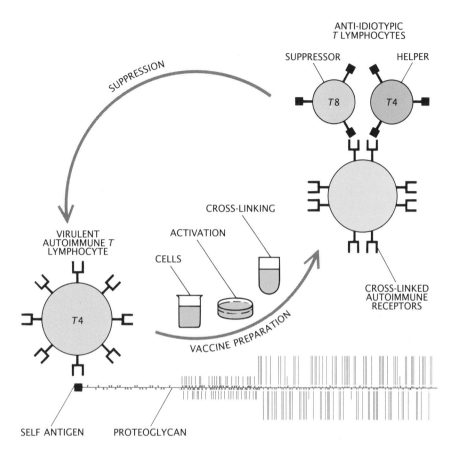

Figure 8.7 POSSIBLE MECHANISM of the vaccine against adjuvant arthritis. The critical cells are the virulent autoimmune T4 cells—with receptors for proteoglycan—that are removed from arthritic rats. Preparation of the vaccine entails aggregating the receptors, a process that increases their potency. When they are injected into other rats suffering from adjuvant arthritis, the aggregated receptors evoke anti-idiotypic T4 and T8 cells. The T8 cells are "suppressors" that may inhibit the proliferation of the autoimmune lymphocytes. The T4 cells are "helpers." Helpers facilitate the growth of B and T cells; their function in the vaccinated rat is not as yet understood.

of the T lymphocytes into a mass; this was accomplished either physically (through hydrostatic pressure) or chemically (through agents that cross-link cell-surface receptors). Apparently, aggregating the receptors makes them much more potent in generat-

Figure 8.6 VACCINE AGAINST AUTOIMMUNITY was developed by the author and his colleagues. Three groups of rats were inoculated with an adjuvant containing M. tuberculosis; all three developed adjuvant arthritis. Autoimmune cells from the lymph nodes of one group (a) were removed, processed to increase their immunogenic effects and then injected into the second group (b). After inoculation the vaccinated group experienced remission of the disease. The untreated group (c) developed chronic arthritis.

ing anti-idiotypic lymphocytes. Even more striking, the vaccine also serves as a form of therapy: rats receiving cross-linked T lymphocytes taken from other sick rats quickly underwent permanent remission of their autoimmune disease.

It is not yet known exactly how T-cell vaccination induces resistance to the autoimmune process, but some suggestive data are being accumulated (see Figure 8.7). Our most recent work confirms that in response to vaccination anti-idiotypic T lymphocytes emerge that specifically recognize the receptors of the disease-causing T cells. The anti-idiotypic lymphocytes include both cells with the T4 marker and those with T8. The T4 cells are helpers and the T8 cells are suppressors, which inhibit the growth of clones of other lymphocytes. We do not know which type is responsible for resisting the autoimmune disease. It is conceivable that the two groups work in concert to regulate the lymphocytes that cause the autoimmune disease.

The effectiveness of *T*-lymphocyte vaccination in activating lymphocytes capable of modulating autoimmunity is certainly compatible with the general idea of a Jernian network. Our observations, however, by no means establish the physiological role of the network proposed by Jerne; much more work will be required for that. Yet the work done so far has established that the border between the self and the external world is not nearly as clear as was once thought. Self-recognition is not merely a sin punished by autoimmune disease, as Burnet and others believed. On the contrary, it is central to health as well as to illness. The immune system is much more complex than it seemed when immunologists thought it perceived only the external world. That knowledge may ultimately be of very real help in easing the pain of autoimmune disease.

Adoptive Immunotherapy for Cancer

*Also called cell-transfer therapy, it is one
of a new class of approaches being developed to strengthen
the innate ability of the immune system to fight cancer*

• • •

Steven A. Rosenberg
May, 1990

In 1968, when I was a surgical resident at a Boston hospital, I admitted a 63-year-old man complaining of abdominal pain characteristic of a gallstone attack. I then participated in the surgery to remove his gallbladder. It was a routine case, except for one extraordinary feature.

Twelve years earlier the man had come to the same hospital with abdominal trouble of a different kind. He had undergone surgery for stomach cancer. The tumor in the stomach was excised to ease his discomfort, but as often occurs, the cancer had spread to his liver, where it could not be removed. The man was sent home without treatment, presumably to die within several months. Unexpectedly, when he returned to the hospital for evaluation three months later, he was actually gaining strength. He continued to improve and soon stopped returning. Nothing more was heard from him until we operated on his gallbladder more than a decade later, at which point we found that all evidence of his cancer was gone. The cancer had disappeared.

The spontaneous disappearance of cancer is one of the rarest events in medicine and is often cited as evidence that the immune system—the body's main natural defense against viruses and other "foreign invaders" (including transplanted organs) —can sometimes mount an attack against cancer. Such evidence has spurred many investigators, including myself, to seek immunotherapies for cancer: treatments designed to enhance the native ability of the immune system to eliminate cancer cells. What is characteristic and dangerous about cancer cells is, of course, that they divide uncontrollably and can break off from the original tumor to establish growths (metastases) in other tissues.

During the past 10 years my colleagues and I at the National Cancer Institute have developed experimental immunotherapies for cancer. The treatments have led to the regression of advanced cancer in some patients whose tumors had failed to respond to other regimens.

In my laboratory we concentrate on what is called adoptive immunotherapy, or cell-transfer therapy. We remove cells involved in immune defense from a cancer patient and either "educate" the cells to react against the cancer or else enhance their native ability to kill cancer cells. We then return the immune-system cells to the bloodstream. In combination with the transfer of immune-system cells, or alone, we also administer molecules that are important in the immune response. With these molecules, which can be generated in quantity by recombinant-DNA technology, we attempt to stimulate anticancer activity directly in the body's immune-system cells. Several versions of our treatments are now available at many cancer-treatment centers, and we are intensively studying other versions we hope will be more effective.

Many difficulties remain. Immunotherapy can be complex, costly and associated with potentially severe side effects. Still, cell-transfer therapy and other immunotherapies for cancer are gaining a place beside the three traditional approaches: surgery to remove discrete masses, radiation to shrink or kill localized cancers that are not amenable to surgery and chemotherapy (the systemic injection of drugs to destroy cancerous growths throughout the body).

The need for new treatments is profound. Alone or together, surgery, radiation and chemotherapy cure cancer in almost half of the people in whom it develops. But the incidence of cancer, and thus the number of deaths, remains high. The disease arises in one of every four individuals. One in six people in the U.S. and Europe will die of cancer; in 1988 alone, cancer claimed in excess of 485,000 American lives, more than all who died in World War II and the Vietnam War combined.

Immunotherapy is a particularly appealing addition to the existing treatments in part because, like chemotherapy, it can be delivered systemically to combat metastases. What is more, the immune system is selective: it normally attacks only diseased cells, ignoring healthy ones. Hence, immunotherapies might be devised that are more cancer-specific than chemotherapies, which often kill dividing cells somewhat indiscriminately.

The idea of fighting cancer by unleashing the latent powers of the patient's own immune system is not new. Early in the 20th century some physicians attempted this feat by injecting patients with killed bacteria. Other workers, seeking to activate a cancer-specific response, injected patients with their own cancer cells. These approaches met with little success. Recent developments in immunology have, however, produced a vastly improved picture of how the immune system functions and, together with progress in genetic engineering, have yielded new leads for therapy.

It is now clear that the immune response involves the integrated action of an army of different cell types, including such white blood cells as monocytes, macrophages, eosinophils, basophils and lymphocytes. The cells of the immune system differ from those of other organs in that they are not in constant contact with one another; instead they circulate throughout the body, moving freely in and out of the circulatory and lymphatic systems.

The cells each have separate functions, but they interact in many ways and can actually regulate one another's activities. The commander and also the predominant foot soldier of this army is the lymphocyte. There are two major subclasses of lymphocyte—B cells and T cells—and these lymph cells account for the specificity of the immune response.

B cells govern the humoral, or antibody-mediated, arm of the immune response, which neutralizes bacteria and other invaders. Each B cell is able to recognize only a single antigen: a molecule that identifies a bacterium or other invader as "nonself." Activated B cells secrete circulating antibodies that bind to antigens or antigen-bearing targets and mark them for destruction by other components of the immune system.

The T cells direct what is called cell-mediated immunity: the destruction by cells of the immune system of foreign tissues or infected cells. There are a variety of T cells, including "helper" and "suppressor" cells, which modulate the immune response, and cytotoxic (or "killer") cells, which can kill abnormal cells directly. As is true of B cells, each T cell bears receptors for only a single antigen. A T cell that recognizes and binds a unique antigen displayed on the surface of another cell becomes activated: it can multiply, and if it is a cytotoxic cell, it can kill the bound cell. Cancer cells sometimes display antigens not found on healthy cells, and so they can potentially activate T cells carrying receptors for those antigens.

Discoveries made in the 1970's and 1980's further revealed that the cells of the immune system often control one another's activities by secreting small amounts of potent hormones known as cytokines. These newly identified proteins, which include lymphokines (the hormone products of lymphocytes) and monokines (the products of monocytes and macrophages), differ from classic hormones such as insulin in that they normally act locally and do not circulate in the blood.

The new understanding of the immune system led my research group to pursue various lines of investigation into immunotherapy. Hoping to harness the specificity of lymphocytes, we took on the major research challenge of developing adoptive immunotherapy with those cells. We are also studying the effects of delivering one or more cytokines to patients, in an attempt to enhance the cancer-fighting activity of lymphocytes circulating in the body.

The major obstacle to the initial development of the cell-transfer approach for the treatment of human cancer was our inability to isolate from cancer patients, and to expand to large numbers, lymphocytes that have activity against cancer. The potential value of cell-transfer therapy had nonetheless been suggested by studies in animals.

In animals it is possible to raise immune-system cells with reactivity against tumors by repeated immunization of the animals with tumor cells. Indeed, in the late 1960's, Peter Alexander of the Chester Beatty Research Institute in London and Alexander Fefer of the University of Washington showed that the intravenous delivery of lymphocytes from immunized mice into tumor-bearing mice of the same inbred strain could mediate the regression of tumors. (Because the inbred animals are genetically and immunologically identical, the recipient's immune system does not sense that the lymphocytes come from another animal and so does not destroy them.) No feasible way to raise lymphocytes for application in humans had been found, however.

My own first attempts at cell-transfer therapy for humans were born of desperation. In 1968, shortly after encountering the patient whose stomach cancer had disappeared spontaneously, I obtained a unit of blood from him and infused it into another man who also had stomach cancer and was close to death. This transfusion had no effect on the second patient's disease. Similar attempts by other physicians were likewise unsuccessful.

Later I treated a series of cancer patients by delivering lymphocytes derived from pigs immunized against the patients' cancer. The patients were not harmed by the large numbers of pig lymphocytes, but neither were they helped. Thus, although cancer treatments based on the transfer of lymphocytes remained theoretically attractive, the impossibility of isolating and growing the number of cells needed for successful treatment paralyzed progress.

A discovery made in 1976 offered new encouragement. Robert C. Gallo and his colleagues at the National Cancer Institute described a molecule that was originally called T cell growth factor and is now known as interleukin-2 (IL-2). This cytokine is pro-

duced by helper T cells and causes both those cells and antigen-stimulated cytotoxic T cells to replicate (see Chapter 5, "Interleukin-2," by Kendall A. Smith).

The discovery of interleukin-2 and the subsequent introduction of methods for growing abundant clones of T cells in culture with the cytokine suggested a new option. I thought that if my colleagues and I could isolate from a patient even a small number of T cells reactive against the individual's tumor, we might be able to expand the lymphocytes in the laboratory to produce the quantities needed for cell-transfer therapy.

If we were ever to test the ability of such cultured cells to mount an attack against a patient's cancer, we would first have to demonstrate that the injected cells retained their original properties and that they would evoke a strong anticancer response in animals. Therefore, while we sought ways to identify tumor-sensitive T cells in humans, we simultaneously conducted several animal studies of cultured lymphocytes.

In 1981 Maury Rosenstein, a postdoctoral fellow working in my laboratory, demonstrated that cultured T cells injected into mice did indeed maintain the ability to recognize antigen: they accelerated the specific rejection of skin grafts. Within about a year Timothy J. Eberlein, a surgical resident, and I demonstrated that cultured cells could induce the regression of widespread, metastasized cancer in mice.

In this work we extended an approach that had been exploited successfully by Fefer and his co-workers. Fefer's group had induced a lymphoma to form in the abdominal cavity of mice. They had then achieved regression of the tumor by placing cultured T cells from immunized mice in the cavity as well. Eberlein injected cells derived from the same lymphoma into the footpad of mice, waited for the disease to metastasize and then injected cultured T cells from immunized mice into a vein.

We found that the treatment could cause complete regression not only of the tumor growing in the footpad but also of cancer that had spread to the blood and lymph nodes. This result was quite important because it meant that the cultured T cells did not have to be delivered directly to the cancer; after the T cells were injected into the bloodstream, they could find cancer cells on their own.

Later studies by John H. Donohue, another surgical resident in my laboratory, showed that the administration of interleukin-2 simultaneously with the cultured T cells enhanced the antitumor effects of the cell-transfer therapy, inducing cancer regression with fewer T cells. The cytokine probably helped by causing the transferred cells to multiply in the body.

These successes were heartening, but we continued to be stymied by the problem of isolating T cells with antitumor activity from people. Eventually an unexpected finding, made in the course of tackling that problem, led to our first adoptive immunotherapy for human cancer.

The new approach grew out of the discovery in 1980 that interleukin-2 had an unusual activity. Ilana Yron, a postdoctoral fellow, and I reasoned that if the body was mounting an immune response against a cancer, the tumor itself would probably have the highest concentration of tumor-specific lymphocytes. Working with Paul J. Spiess, a biologist in my laboratory, she therefore cultured tumor cells with interleukin-2, aiming to expand and isolate the population of lymphocytes specific for that particular tumor. To their surprise, they found that within three or four days, even before the lymphocytes could multiply, cancer cells next to the white blood cells in the culture appeared to die. It seemed interleukin-2 had an activity not identified before: it could actually stimulate certain lymphocytes to recognize and kill cancer cells.

My colleagues' discovery raised the exciting possibility that we might not need to identify lymphocytes already activated against a patient's cancer; we might be able to induce quiescent cells to attack. Follow-up studies confirmed that we could. When Yron and Spiess exposed lymphocytes from the spleen of healthy mice to interleukin-2, the treated lymphocytes killed tumor cells. Then Michael T. Lotze, a surgical resident, and I extended the work to humans. We showed that exposure to interleukin-2 enabled lymphocytes from the blood of healthy people to kill a variety of human cancer cells in vitro—including those from melanoma (a skin cancer), colon cancer and sarcomas (cancers of connective tissues). The activated cells, which we later named lymphokine-activated killer (LAK) cells, did not harm normal cells.

The pedigree of the cells was another surprise. When Elizabeth A. Grimm joined my laboratory as a postdoctoral fellow and examined the LAK cells in detail, she found that they were not cytotoxic T cells or indeed any kind of T cell. Nor were they B cells. They were derived from the "null" population that constitutes only about 5 percent of all circulating lymphocytes. These cells, ubiquitous in mammals, appear to be part of a primitive immunosurveillance mechanism that can eliminate cancerous or otherwise altered cells nonspecifically, without first having to recognize a particular antigen. The ability of the LAK cells to kill a variety of tumor types in vitro suggested that their injection into patients with cancer might be beneficial.

The idea had to be tested in animals before it could be tested in people. In 1984, in my laboratory's first successful immunotherapy experiments with LAK cells, Amitabha Mazumder, a pediatric oncology fellow, injected the cells intravenously into mice whose melanoma had given rise to lung metastases. We found after two weeks that the lungs of the treated animals contained far less cancer than did the lungs of the untreated subjects in a control group. Next James J. Mulé, a postdoctoral fellow, and I quickly showed that administration of interleukin-2 along with the LAK cells enhanced the antitumor activity of the cells, much as it had earlier when the cytokine was delivered with T cells derived from immunized animals.

Other investigations revealed that interleukin-2 improved the therapeutic effectiveness of the LAK treatment by stimulating the cells to multiply in the body. Stephen E. Ettinghausen, a surgical resident, and I discovered that infused LAK cells divide in the organs of mice that receive both the cells and interleukin-2 but do not divide when the cells are administered alone. The series of studies suggested that LAK cells could travel in the body to cancers in animals. Under the influence of administered interleukin-2, they also proliferate at tumor sites and destroy cancer cells there.

Given that interleukin-2 improved the effects of LAK treatment, we naturally wondered whether injecting mice with the cytokine by itself could activate the anticancer properties of lymphocytes in the body. If so, large doses would probably be required, because the kidneys rapidly destroy circulating interleukin-2. When the gene for interleukin-2 was cloned and large amounts of the gene product became available, we ran the experiment. Indeed, very high doses of the substance alone did have antitumor effects in mice, although the results were not as impressive as when LAK cells were also administered.

By early in 1984, after doing preliminary clinical trials with killer lymphocytes that were activated by noncytokine immune stimulators, we were ready to undertake phase I trials to establish in humans the safety and the highest tolerated doses of LAK cells and interleukin-2. Because neither LAK cells nor interleukin-2 had ever been administered to patients, we could not begin with the combined therapy; instead we tested each substance separately. Each of the subjects in these and subsequent trials suffered from advanced cancer that had failed to respond to all standard therapies; none were expected to survive more than several months.

We treated six patients with activated LAK cells obtained by isolating the patients' own lymphocytes and then incubating the cells with interleukin-2. Typically we isolate the lymphocytes from circulating blood (see Figure 9.1). Thirty-nine other patients

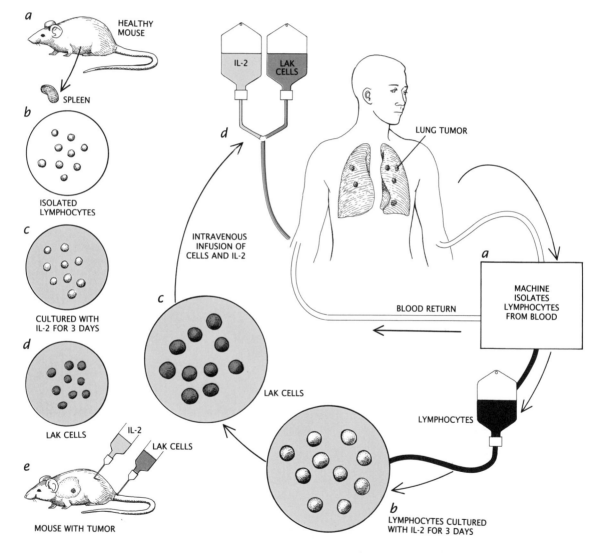

Figure 9.1 LAK CELLS are an experimental anticancer weapon. For study in mice (*left*), production begins with the removal of the spleen from healthy animals (*a*). The lymphocytes in the spleen are isolated (*b*) and cultured for three days with interleukin-2 (*c*), which causes null cells to become LAK cells (*d*), which can recognize and attack a variety of cancers. LAK cells, together with interleukin-2, are injected into tumor-bearing mice (*e*). For study in humans (*right*), lymphocytes are isolated from the bloodstream (*a*) and cultured with IL-2 (*b*) to generate LAK cells (*c*). When patients are treated (*d*), about 50 billion LAK cells are infused intravenously along with IL-2.

were treated with varying doses of interleukin-2 by itself. None of the patients showed any detectable antitumor response. Later in 1984, after reviewing our data, the Food and Drug Administration gave us permission to test the combination of LAK cells and interleukin-2 as a treatment for patients with advanced cancer.

One of the first patients in the new trial was a 29-year-old nurse from Florida who had melanoma that had spread throughout her body, including to her arms, thighs, back and buttocks (see Figure 9.2). Some tumors had been surgically removed, but others had appeared and had not responded to treatment with the drug interferon. We began her combination therapy with LAK cells and interleukin-2 in November, 1984. During the next three months all of her cancer disappeared. Today, more than five years later, she remains free of the disease.

Her case, which we reported along with 24 others in a 1985 paper in the *New England Journal of Medicine*, was the first demonstration that a therapy aimed at strengthening the activity of a patient's own lymphocytes could induce cancer regression. To date, we have studied more than 150 patients with advanced cancer, the majority of whom had melanoma or kidney cancer. (In most patients the original tumor or tumors had been removed, and in all patients the cancer had metastasized.) We have achieved complete tumor regression in about 10 percent of the patients with melanoma and 10 percent of patients with kidney cancer; the tumor mass decreased by at least 50 percent in another 10 per-

cent of those with melanoma and 25 percent with kidney cancer. We have also achieved complete or partial regression of advanced cancer in patients with non-Hodgkin's lymphoma and colon cancer. As for specific tissues, cancers have been reduced or eliminated from the lung, liver, bone, skin and subcutaneous tissue.

The therapy seems to work in people much as it does in mice. When we removed cancerous nodules from patients receiving the immunotherapy, we found extensive infiltration by lymphocytes along with many dead tumor cells. It appears that LAK cells and other lymphocytes make their way to tumors and, under the influence of the continuous administration of interleukin-2, divide there, causing cancer regression. Other studies have since shown that high doses of interleukin-2 administered alone can also induce cancer regression in some patients. Whether this treatment is as effective as the combined therapy remains to be determined (see Figure 9.3).

Immunotherapy based on the administration of LAK cells plus interleukin-2 or in some cases of interleukin-2 alone is thus a treatment that can help about 20 percent of patients with certain advanced cancers. But its success comes at a price: there can be side effects. The proliferation of lymphocytes in tissues can interfere with the function of vital organs. The administration of high doses of interleukin-2 leads to the leakage of fluid from the blood into tissues, and weight gain from the fluid is common. Less commonly, the accumulating fluid im-

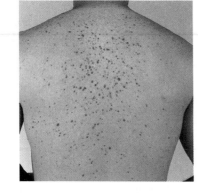 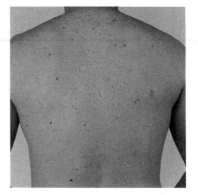

Figure 9.2 MELANOMA TUMORS that had spread across a patient's back (*left*) disappeared after LAK cells and interleukin-2 were infused (*right*). Cancer regresses fully in about 10 percent of patients with advanced melanoma or kidney cancer given this treatment.

Cancer Diagnosis	TREATMENT WITH LAK CELLS AND IL-2				TREATMENT WITH IL-2 ALONE			
	Number of Patients	Complete Regression	Partial Regression (At Least 50% of Tumor Mass)	Complete or Partial Regression	Number of Patients	Complete Regression	Partial Regression (At Least 50% of Tumor Mass)	Complete or Partial Regression
KIDNEY	72	8	17	25 (35%)	54	4	8	12 (22%)
MELANOMA	48	4	6	10 (21%)	42	0	10	10 (24%)
COLORECTAL	30	1	4	5 (17%)	12	0	0	0
NON-HODGKIN'S LYMPHOMA	7	1	3	4 (57%)	11	0	0	0
SARCOMA	6	0	0	0	—	—	—	—
LUNG	5	0	0	0	—	—	—	—
BREAST	—	—	—	—	3	0	0	0
OTHER	9	0	0	0	8	0	0	0
TOTAL	177	14	30	44 (25%)	130	4	18	22 (17%)

Figure 9.3 MORE THAN 300 PATIENTS with advanced cancers have been treated either with LAK cells and interleukin-2 or with interleukin-2 alone, which by itself can cause some cancer regression in both mice and humans. In mice the combination therapy is more effective than interleukin-2 alone, but more data are needed before a similar conclusion can be drawn for humans.

pairs lung function and thereby impedes the delivery of oxygen to tissues. Very occasionally patients die from the effects of the interleukin-2, but the mortality—about 1 percent—is less than that associated with almost any systemic chemotherapy prescribed today for people with advanced cancer. In the remaining 99 percent of our patients, the side effects disappear rapidly once treatment is completed.

Treatment with LAK cells and interleukin-2 or with interleukin-2 alone is still experimental. In 1987, however, the FDA gave approval for federally designated Comprehensive Cancer Centers and Clinical Cancer Research Centers across the country to administer such therapy to patients with advanced melanoma or kidney cancer.

Our encouraging results with LAK cells led us to search for cells that were even more potent against cancer. We have recently found such cells. We discovered them about four years ago, after resuming our efforts to identify cells already activated against a patient's specific cancer. We again postulated that if the immune system were aroused against a cancer, the tumor site should have the highest concentration of cancer-sensitive lympho-cytes. We therefore developed new techniques for isolating lymphocytes from tumors.

In one method we surgically removed a small tumor from an animal, enzymatically digested it to separate the cells and then cultured the cells with interleukin-2 for several weeks. During that time, what we call tumor-infiltrating lymphocytes (TIL's) —lymphocytes in the tumor—multiplied under the influence of the interleukin-2. LAK cells generally stop proliferating after about 10 days, but other lymphocytes capable of killing the tumor continued to grow vigorously and eventually replaced the tumor. We then analyzed these proliferating TIL's and studied their effects in animals.

The TIL's that overran the culture turned out to be classic cytotoxic T cells. Unlike LAK cells, they had the specificity we initially sought. On exposure to tumor cells in laboratory dishes, such TIL's often kill only the cells of the tumors from which they are derived and no others. In fact, they represent the best available evidence that at least some humans with cancer do indeed mount a specific immunologic reaction against their tumor.

When we injected our newly isolated cytotoxic TIL's into mice, we found that, on a cell-for-cell basis, they were from 50 to 100 times more effective than LAK cells in causing regression of established tumors—a finding we reported in 1986. That is, if 100 million LAK cells were needed to produce a 50 percent regression in an animal's cancer, only from one million to two million TIL's would be required to achieve the same degree of success. We also found that the TIL's were more effective than LAK cells at eliminating cancer in mice with widespread tumors.

It was not long before we began studying the efficacy of TIL therapy in patients (see Figure 9.4). We obtained the TIL's by surgically removing a tumor nodule approximately the size of a small plum from patients, in most cases under local anesthesia. From the nodule we obtained about 50 million tumor cells; we then cultured them with interleukin-2 until they all died and were replaced by a rich supply of multiplying TIL's. Then approxi-

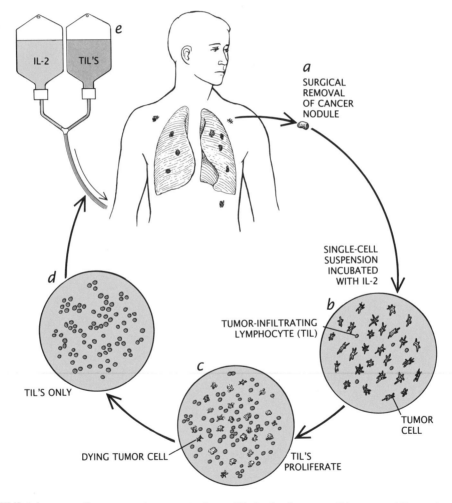

Figure 9.4 TIL'S take a month or more to generate for administration to patients. After a nodule of cancerous tissue is removed from a patient (*a*), cells in the nodule are separated from one another by enzymes and then cultured with interleukin-2 (*b*). Under the influence of the IL-2, lymphocytes scattered throughout the tumor—the TIL's (*blue*)—begin to proliferate rapidly and to attack the cancer cells (*c*). After a total of 30 to 45 days, the lymphocytes in the culture completely replace the tumor cells (*d*). Two-hundred billion of these replacement TIL's are then infused into the patient along with additional IL-2 (*e*).

mately 200 billion of these cells were delivered intravenously, along with interleukin-2.

Data on the first 20 patients treated by this approach appeared in the *New England Journal* in December, 1988, almost exactly three years from the report of the first successful trials of LAK cells in humans. All the subjects had melanoma. Fifteen had never before been treated with interleukin-2, and in nine of these the melanoma regressed by at least 50 percent (see Figure 9.5). The same degree of tumor reduction was also seen in two of the five patients who had received high doses of interleukin-2 in the past but to no avail. Thus, 55 percent of our group responded well to the therapy. In fact, the response rate was more than twice that seen when we gave LAK cells and interleukin-2 to patients with melanoma. We do not yet have a good sense of how long cancer regression will persist on average, although thus far cancers have remained in complete or partial remission for from several months to more than a year.

How do the TIL's work? Studies of radioactively labeled cells have shown that some fraction of the cells travel to cancer sites and accumulate there in the days following TIL infusion. Analyses of messenger RNA, the templates for proteins in a cell, suggest that the TIL's destroy tumor cells not only by direct contact but also through production of cytokines capable of mediating tumor-cell killing.

Because TIL therapy includes infusions of interleukin-2, it produces much the same set of side effects as does LAK therapy. Yet the TIL's require less interleukin-2 to remain alive and active in the body, and so in the future we may be able to administer less interleukin-2 and thereby reduce the side effects.

Both LAK and TIL therapy exploit cells that nature has provided to the patient, and each is helpful for some people with some cancers. Might the innate therapeutic properties of those cells be improved by making small, carefully designed changes in their genes? My laboratory is collaborating with two others to create and test such "designer lymphocytes." The heads of those laboratories are R. Michael Blaese of the National Cancer Institute and W. French Anderson of the National Heart, Lung and Blood Institute, who have been developing gene-transfer techniques in the hope of eventually correcting inborn genetic defects in humans.

In 1988 Blaese, Anderson and I devised a two-phase strategy for testing genetically engineered lymphocytes in cancer patients. In the first phase we planned to introduce a foreign gene encoding a protein that would simply be a marker, helping us to determine the fate of TIL's in patients and to recover the cells for further analysis. We settled on a

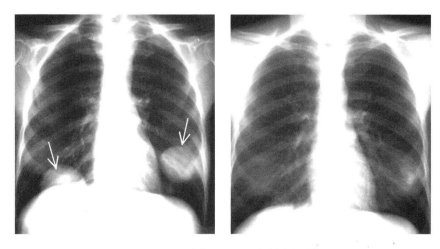

Figure 9.5 X-RAY IMAGE made in October, 1987 (*left*), shows that melanoma had spread to a patient's lung (*arrows*). By December, after the patient was treated with TIL's and interleukin-2, most of the cancer had disappeared (*right*). Of 20 patients thus treated for advanced melanoma, 11 had a regression of at least 50 percent of their tumor mass.

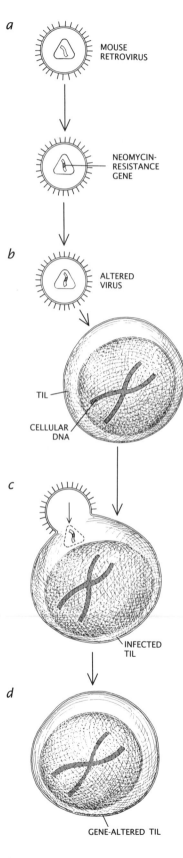

Figure 9.6 INSERTION of a foreign gene into TIL's is accomplished by a mouse retrovirus. In order to make the only genetically altered TIL's administered to patients thus far, workers replace retroviral genes crucial to viral replication with a gene encoding a protein that can render cells resistant to the lethal effects of the antibiotic neomycin (*a*). The altered virus is cultured with TIL's (*b*) so that the virus can infect the cells (*c*) and install its genetic material in the cellular DNA (*d*). The foreign gene replicates whenever the infected TIL's replicate. Because altered TIL's express the foreign gene, they are uniquely resistant to neomycin and hence are readily distinguishable from all other cells in the body.

gene for a protein that normally makes bacteria resistant to a form of the antibiotic neomycin. Because TIL's would be the only cells in the body producing this protein, the substance would give us an easy way to identify the transferred lymphocytes. In this phase, which is now under way, we have performed the first successful introduction of foreign genes into human beings.

In the second phase, not yet begun, we planned to insert a gene into TIL's that we thought could enhance their therapeutic potency. Among the candidates we are still considering are the genes for the cytokines tumor necrosis factor and alpha interferon (both of which are known to have antitumor properties) or perhaps even the gene for interleukin-2 itself.

Our proposal for accomplishing the first phase was straightforward. We would remove a tumor deposit from a patient with advanced melanoma and grow TIL's as before. After about two weeks, when all the cancer cells were dead, we would take a small sample of the TIL's and introduce the neomycin-resistance gene. Although there are many techniques that can be exploited for introducing genes into mammalian cells, only one of these, which depends on the activity of retroviruses (RNA viruses), is efficient enough to be practical for our purposes. We selected a mouse retrovirus that was genetically engineered so that it could introduce the gene of interest into the TIL's but could not itself reproduce: all of the gene sequences required for viral replication were removed and replaced by the neomycin-resistance gene (see Figure 9.6).

Once the alteration of the TIL's was accomplished by the retroviruses, the altered human cells would then be multiplied in parallel with the original TIL's. After verifying that the new gene was inserted and expressed as protein in the TIL's, we would infuse the altered cells along with nontreated cells into patients. (The unaltered cells were included in order to provide the desired therapeutic doses of TIL's.) Interleukin-2 would be administered as well.

Because of the newness of the gene-transfer technology and the fact that no gene-transfer studies had ever been authorized in humans, the government carefully evaluated the practical and ethical questions raised by our proposed trial. We initiated the review process on June 20, 1988, by submitting our protocol to the Investigational Review Boards of the National Institutes of Health. We received approval from James Wyngaarden, then the director of

the institutes, on January 19, 1989. The agency would permit us to begin a clinical trial of 10 patients with advanced melanoma, all of whom had a life expectancy of 90 days or less.

During the intervening months the institutes' Biosafety Committee and Recombinant DNA Advisory Committee as well as the FDA had conducted additional reviews. These groups insisted that we demonstrate the ability to insert the marker gene in human TIL's and induce the cells to synthesize the encoded protein. They also required us to show that the TIL's were not significantly altered by the insertion of the gene, that we could detect marked cells in laboratory animals and that there was low risk to the patient and no risk to the public. We satisfied them on all counts. Then, on the day Wyngaarden announced his approval of the trial, a biotechnology activist filed a lawsuit to prevent us from proceeding, claiming the study had not had sufficient review. We were delayed again, but fortunately, the suit was settled quickly.

We treated the first person ever to receive gene-modified cells on May 22, 1989. We plan to report the results on the first five patients receiving these cells by this summer. Within a year we hope to begin studying TIL's genetically altered to have an improved therapeutic effect. The feasibility of exploiting genetically altered TIL's for cancer therapy will probably take several years to determine.

The therapeutic possibilities of genetically altered lymphocytes obviously extend far beyond cancer treatment. The cells may prove to be suitable vehicles for introducing genes that can treat a variety of other diseases in addition to cancer. For instance, genes that direct the production of clotting factors might be introduced into the body for treating hemophilia. Genes that encode the enzyme adenosine deaminase might be exploited to treat severe combined immunodeficiency disease, which makes certain children abnormally susceptible to life-threatening infections.

What was once an intuition is now becoming a reality. Immunotherapy for cancer can be effective. The treatments developed thus far can help only a limited number of patients, have toxic side effects and are complex and cumbersome to perform. But perhaps they are only the beginning. Extensive efforts are under way in laboratories around the world to develop immunotherapy into a practical, effective way to treat human cancer.

MONOCLONAL ANTIBODIES AND THEIR APPLICATION

. . .

Introduction

The random structure generator of lymphocytes and antigen-driven selection provides an efficient mechanism for the development of antibodies of any desired specificity. The use of antibodies to detect virtually any structure has long been recognized as having enormous value. Indeed, antibody assays have been the preferred method to measure small amounts of proteins and other substances. Solomon Berson and Rosalyn Yalow demonstrated the power of this approach with their development of radioimmunoassays, initially for insulin in blood. Subsequently, radioimmunoassays and related methods such as enzyme-lined immunosorbent assays have been used in virtually every situation where simplicity, sensitivity and specificity is required for measurement of proteins and other substances. Yalow was recognized for this major achievement with the award of the Nobel Prize in physiology or medicine in 1977.

Although antibodies obtained from the serum of immunized animals have been enormously valuable, such antisera often offer unexpected problems. This stems from the fact that they are actually a collection of a large number of distinct antibodies, each with a characteristic specificity. The population of antibodies as a whole is, of course, specific for the immunogen but each of the component antibodies has a range of cross-reactivities that provide the antiserum with the potential of a wide range of unanticipated specificities. Furthermore, different antisera obtained as a result of immunization with the same antigen can vary so that different lots of these reagents may have quite different properties.

The introduction of the monoclonal antibody technique has extended the potential of immunologic specificity into new arenas. Chapter 10, "Monoclonal Antibodies," by Cesar Milstein, describes the development of this technique, for which he and his colleague Georges Köhler received the Nobel Prize in physiology or medicine in 1984. The technique is based on the fact that individual antibody-secreting cells produce a single species of antibodies. By fusing precursors of such antibody-producing cells with a myeloma cell line (a malignant antibody-producing cell line), one can obtain immortalized cells capable of producing but a single antibody. Indeed, the myeloma cell line used as the fusion partner has been selected for the loss of the capacity to produce its own immunoglobulin, so that the antibody of the normal fusion partner is the only one made by the hybridoma resulting from the fusion (hybridization) of the normal cell and the myeloma cell line.

In principle, through the use of appropriate immunization procedures and of techniques to select hybridomas secreting antibodies of the desired specificity, molecules highly specific for virtually any antigen can be obtained. Furthermore, one can use such an approach to produce antibodies specific for a given protein present in a complex mixture and thus to use the resultant antibodies for the purification and characterization of the immunizing protein.

Chapter 11, "Catalytic Antibodies," by Richard A. Lerner and Alfonso Tramontano, deals with another exciting application of the monoclonal antibody technology. It describes the fact that antibodies directed at epitopes found on transitional states in a chemical reaction can act as catalysts to enable such reactions to proceed much more rapidly, just as enzymes do. The fact that monoclonal antibodies could be made against virtually any structure, provided one can obtain an immunogen that contains the epitope and can devise a selection strategy allowing one to identify the appropriate hybridoma, holds the promise that antibodies can be obtained that are capable of catalyzing reactions for which natural enzymes do not exist. Efforts to extend this technique into a variety of types of chemical reactions are underway with very promising results.

"Immunotoxins," Chapter 12, by R. John Collier and Donald A. Kaplan, describes a second area in which monoclonal antibodies may make possible a dream of immunologists and of chemotherapists. It is the concept of the "magic bullet," the therapeutic agent endowed with the specificity to identify and thus act only on a particular tissue or a particular set of cells. Efforts to use this approach with conventional antibodies as the targeting agent, covalently associated with a chemotherapeutic drug or a toxin, were largely unsuccessful because the specificity of the antibodies was not sufficient to allow precise targeting and because means to improve the characteristics of the antibody by genetic engineering did not exist. The development of the monoclonal antibody technique and progress in the understanding of the structure and mode of action of many toxins now makes the magic bullet or immunotoxin concept one with real promise. A variety of toxins have been covalently associated with monoclonal antibodies specific for markers that are found on tumor cells. To make this approach a practical one, it is necessary to have antibodies or other targeting structures (such as growth factors) that are highly specific for the target, usually a tumor; the natural targeting structures of the toxin must be removed or disabled without diminishing the action of the toxin, and the capacity of the toxin to gain access to the cellular compartment in which it is active must be ensured. Great progress has been made in each of these areas so that immunotoxins may prove to be a reality for treatment of tumors and for other uses in the not-too-distant future.

Monoclonal Antibodies

Cells that secrete antibodies can be made immortal by fusing them with tumor cells and cloning the hybrids. Each clone is a long-term source of substantial quantities of a single highly specific antibody.

. . .

Cesar Milstein
October, 1980

When a foreign substance enters the body of a vertebrate animal or is injected into it, one aspect of the immune response is the secretion by plasma cells of antibodies: immunoglobulin molecules with combining sites that recognize the shape of particular determinants on the surface of the foreign substance, or antigen, and bind to them. The combination of antibody with antigen sets in train processes that can neutralize and eliminate the foreign substance. Quite apart from the natural function of antibodies in the immune response they have long been an important tool for investigators, who capitalize on their specificity to identify or label particular molecules or cells and to separate them from a mixture.

The antibody response to a typical antigen is highly heterogeneous. There are perhaps a million different lines of B lymphocytes, the precursors of plasma cells, in the spleen of a mouse or a man. All are derived from a common stem cell, but each line develops an independent capacity to make an antibody that recognizes a different antigenic determinant. When an animal is injected with an immunizing agent, it responds by making diverse antibodies directed against different antigen molecules on the injected substance and different determinants on a single antigen, and even different antibodies that fit, more or less well, a single determinant. It is next to impossible to separate the various antibodies, and so conventional antiserums contain mixtures of antibodies, and the mixtures vary from animal to animal (see Figure 10.1).

Each antibody is made, however, by a different line of lymphocytes and their derived plasma cells. What if one could pluck out one such cell making a single specific antibody and grow it in culture? The single cell's progeny, or clone, would be a source of large amounts of identical antibody against a single antigenic determinant: a monoclonal antibody. Unfortunately antibody-secreting cells cannot be maintained in a culture medium.

There are malignant tumors of the immune system called myelomas, however, whose rapidly proliferating cells produce large amounts of abnormal immunoglobulins called myeloma proteins. A tumor is itself an immortal clone of cells descended from a single progenitor, and so myeloma cells can be cultured indefinitely, and all the immunoglobulins they secrete are identical in chemical structure. They are in effect monoclonal antibodies, but there

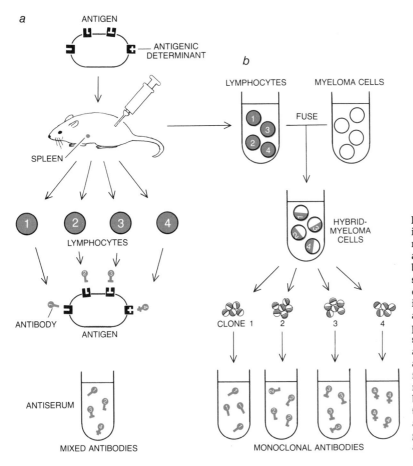

Figure 10.1 IMMUNE RESPONSE is initiated (*a*) when an antigen molecule carrying several different antigenic determinants enters the body of an animal. The immune system responds: lines of *B* lymphocytes proliferate, each secreting an immunoglobulin molecule that fits a single antigenic determinant (or a part of it). A conventional antiserum contains a mixture of these antibodies. Monoclonal antibodies are derived by fusing lymphocytes from the spleen with malignant myeloma cells (*b*). Individual hybrid cells are cloned, and each of the clones secretes a monoclonal antibody that specifically fits a single antigenic determinant on the antibody molecule.

is no way to know what antigen they are directed against, nor can one induce myelomas that produce antibody to a specific antigen.

In 1975 my colleagues and I learned how to fuse mouse myeloma cells with lymphocytes from the spleen of mice immunized with a particular antigen. The resulting hybrid-myeloma, or "hybridoma," cells express both the lymphocyte's property of specific-antibody production and the immortal character of the myeloma cells. Such hybrid cells can be manipulated by the techniques applicable to animal cells in permanent culture. Individual hybrid cells can be cloned, and each clone produces large amounts of identical antibody to a single antigenic determinant. The individual clones can be maintained indefinitely, and at any time samples can be grown in culture or injected into animals for the large-scale production of monoclonal antibody. Highly specific monoclonal antibodies produced by

this general method have proved to be a remarkably versatile tool in many areas of biological research and clinical medicine.

Human myelomas have been known to physicians for a long time, but it was not until the early 1960's that the precise nature of myeloma proteins was elucidated by immunologists. Michael Potter of the National Cancer Institute then induced myelomas in mice, and these too produced large amounts of monoclonal immunoglobulins. In spite of much effort, however, it was not possible to induce tumors that could synthesize antibodies to an injected antigen. Leo Sachs, Kenko Horibata, Edwin S. Lennox and Melvin Cohn did succeed in establishing a line of mouse myeloma cells in tissue culture at the Salk Institute for Biological Studies, but the line was then lost. Eventually Horibata and A. W. Harris were able to establish a number of lines, which they distributed to other laboratories. My group at the Medical Research Council Laboratory of Molecular Biology in Cambridge subjected a line derived from one of Potter's tumors to intensive study.

At that time we were not thinking about monoclonal antibodies. We were studying how somatic (body) cells diversify in culture and how mutations modify the combining specificity of antibodies, and the mouse myeloma line was for us simply another appropriate tissue-culture line. By 1973 Richard G. Cotton, David S. Secher and I were able for the first time to produce structural mutants of a mouse myeloma protein secreted by a cultured cell line. That work and parallel investigations by Matthew D. Scharff of the Albert Einstein College of Medicine in New York demonstrated spontaneous mutations in cultured cells that affected the structure of the proteins they manufactured, and also told something about the molecular nature of the mutations and their frequency. The search for mutants was laborious, however, because the proteins made by the parental cells lacked recognizable antibody activity, changes in which would be the most effective indication of slight differences caused by mutations. Clearly what was needed was a cell line that secreted an immunoglobulin exhibiting antibody activity that could be easily assayed. No such line existed.

At that point a lucky circumstance led us to the hybrid-myeloma technique. While we were working on somatic mutations Georges Köhler and I were also following a quite different line of research in an attempt to learn more about the genetic control of the synthesis of antibodies. The synthesis of antibodies is controlled by two sets of genes. One set encodes the "variable" region of the antibody molecule's light and heavy chains, the region that controls antibody specificity; the other set encodes the "constant" region of the chains, the region that is responsible for such effector functions as the binding of complement (a complex of blood-plasma proteins implicated in the immune response), the transport of the antibody molecule across membranes and the binding of the molecule to membranes. Each lymphocyte synthesizes an antibody encoded by a single pair of V (for variable) and C (for constant) genes out of a large repertoire of such genes in the cell, and when there are different alleles, or variant forms, of a V or a C gene on each of the cell's two chromosomes, only the allele on one of the chromosomes is active; the other is excluded.

In 1973 Cotton and I did an experiment to find out if allelic exclusion could be broken and, if it could, what the molecular consequences would be. We fused two myeloma cells, one from a mouse line and one from a rat line. Analysis of the hybrid cells showed that they secreted hybrid molecules consisting of various combinations of the chains synthesized by the parental cells but never a combination of a V region from one animal and a C region from the other. That meant the genes for the V and the C regions must be on the same chromosome. It is now known that the DNA sequences coding for the V and the C regions are separated by introns, or intervening sequences of DNA. The entire stretch of DNA is transcribed into a complementary strand of nuclear RNA. The RNA is processed by cellular enzymes—the intron is excised and the sequences coding for the V and the C regions are spliced together—to make the messenger RNA that is thereupon translated into the protein of the immunoglobulin chain. The hybrid-myeloma experiment, in other words, showed that the splicing of the V and the C sequences takes place within a single molecule of RNA.

This experiment also showed that there was no allelic exclusion in the hybrids, because the information from both parents was "codominantly" expressed by the fused cells. That finding suggested to Köhler and me a possible answer to our need for an antibody-producing cell in the mutation experiment. It occurred to us that it might be possible to fuse a normal lymphocyte or plasma cell with a myeloma cell and thus to immortalize the expression of the plasma cell's specific-antibody secretion. We would be applying the well-established cell-fusion technique to a new purpose, namely to fix in a permanent cell line a function that is normally expressed only in a "terminal" cell: the plasma cell derived from a B lymphocyte stimulated by an antigen.

For our first attempt we chose sheep red blood cells as the immunogen because antibody against such cells is easily detected by an assay developed by Niels Kaj Jerne and Albert Nordin in 1963. We mixed mouse myeloma cells with spleen cells from immunized mice in the presence of an agent that promotes cell fusion, identified successfully fused cells in a selective medium and found that they secreted immunoglobulins from both parents. Some of them secreted antibody against the red blood cells (see Figure 10.2). We were able to isolate clones that secreted single molecular species of that anti-

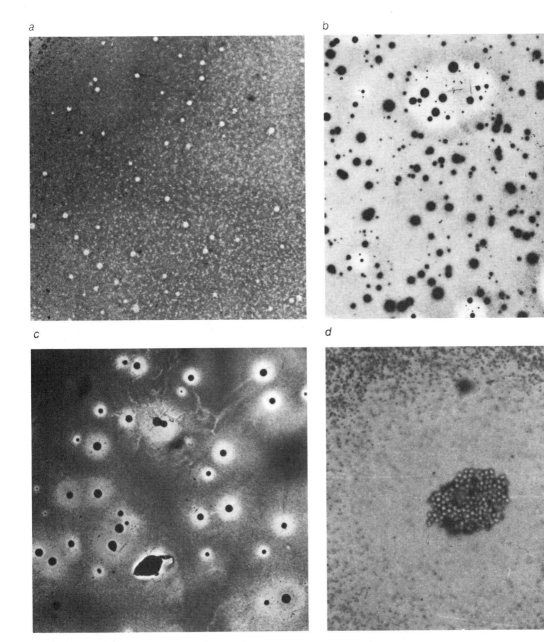

Figure 10.2 ANTIBODY-SECRETING CLONES of hybrid-myeloma cells were first detected by a test for antibodies to sheep red blood cells (srbc). Red cells and antibody-secreting cells are incubated on agar, and complement (a protein complex from blood plasma) is added (*top left*). Antibody diffusing from each secreting cell binds to antigens on nearby blood cells, initiating a complement reaction that kills blood cells, forming a plaque: a clear area (*white spots*) around each secreting cell. Cells from mice immunized with srbc were fused with myeloma cells and plated (*top right*). Hybrid-cell colonies developed (*black spots*). When a layer of srbc was added along with complement, a few hybrid colonies gave rise to plaques (*white areas around colonies*), indicating that they were secreting specific antibody. Individual cells were picked from a colony of antibody-secreting cells and plated thinly (*bottom left*); most of the clones derived from them proved to be secretors of the anti-srbc antibody. A single secreting clone is shown (*bottom right*) with the individual cells of the clone and the area of dead srbc around it.

body, and the clones could be maintained in culture. We had for the first time developed continuous cultures of fused cells secreting a monoclonal antibody of predefined specificity.

After our initial success in 1975 we ran into trouble, and for almost six months the experiments in our laboratory went badly or not at all; Köhler, who had moved to the Basel Institute for Immunology, reported difficulties too. Then Giovanni Galfré came to work in our laboratory and tried various modifications, in particular the use of polyethylene glycol as the fusing agent. It was a depressing period, but it did allow us to optimize the conditions for each step. Eventually the basic problem was discovered: a toxic batch of one of the reagents. Once that fault was remedied, with Jonathan C. Howard and Geoffrey W. Butcher of the Agricultural Research Council Institute of Animal Physiology in Cambridge we achieved a spectacularly successful fusion that produced a series of monoclonal antibodies to rat histocompatibility antigens: the cell-surface markers that establish individual identity and are responsible for the rejection of grafts. Other results began to come in at a rapid pace as we established a standard protocol for the experiments and developed new methods for assaying antibody secretion (see Figure 10.3).

The success of these experiments was enhanced by an unexpected feature. Of the spleen cells we were fusing only perhaps one in 100 was an actively antibody-secreting plasma cell, and yet about one in 10 of our hybrid clones turned out to secrete antibody. That is, we had 10 times as many positive, immortal hybrids as one would expect if immortality were randomly transferred to the heterogeneous spleen-cell population; apparently we were achieving selectivity along with immortality. The explanation for this selectivity is not completely established, but according to recent evidence it probably has two components. On the one hand, secretion seems to be amplified, with lymphocytes that synthesize antibody but do not normally secrete it giving rise to hybrids that both synthesize and secrete antibody. Probably the myeloma parent provides the secreting machinery some antibody producers lack. On the other hand, the conditions under which the fusion takes place apparently make it unlikely that spleen cells other than B lymphocytes will give rise to long-lived hybrids.

When a clone of fused cells has been established, by definition all of the antibody it secretes is genetically derived from a single cell. It is not yet necessarily a monoclonal antibody in the immunological sense of the word, however, because each cell of the hybrid clone has some chromosomes from the myeloma-cell parent and some from the spleen-cell parent and is expressing both sets of chromosomes. Potentially a hybrid cell, instead of producing only the two components of a true monoclonal antibody (one kind of heavy chain and one kind of light chain), can produce two heavy chains and two light ones. We refer to such a cell as HLGK because it secretes the heavy and the light chains of the spleen-cell parent and the corresponding gamma and kappa chains of the myeloma-cell parent. It is in the nature of hybrid cells, particularly in the early stages of proliferation, to lose chromosomes rapidly. In this case the detectable loss is not random: heavy chains (H or G) are usually lost first, and then one or the other of the light chains (L or K) is lost. The HLGK hybrid therefore gives rise to variants whose secretion pattern is HLK or GLK, and these in turn to such variants as HL, HK, LK, L and K.

It is the clone of HL cells, expressing only the heavy chain and the light chain of the specifically immune spleen cell, that one is looking for (although there are reasons for also preserving other variants, notably HK). As one clones it is therefore necessary not only to assay for the specific antibody but also to analyze the immunoglobulin for its type of chain and select a strongly secreting HL (or HK) clone. The selection process can be simplified by choosing a mutant myeloma line that expresses only the light chain (K) and therefore yields HLK hybrids or one that does not express any immunoglobulin and therefore yields an immunologically monoclonal HL hybrid at the outset (see Figure 10.4).

Once the desired clone is selected it can be frozen for long-term storage. At any time a sample of the clone can be injected into animals of the same strain as those that provided the original cells for fusing. The animals develop tumors secreting the specific monoclonal antibody produced by the clone, and the antibody is present in their serum in extremely high concentrations: usually more than 10 milligrams of antibody per milliliter of serum, which in some examples is equivalent to a titer of perhaps a million. Alternatively a sample of the clone can be grown in a mass culture and the antibody can be harvested from the medium.

We have exploited methods similar to the one I have described to produce antibodies to a broad

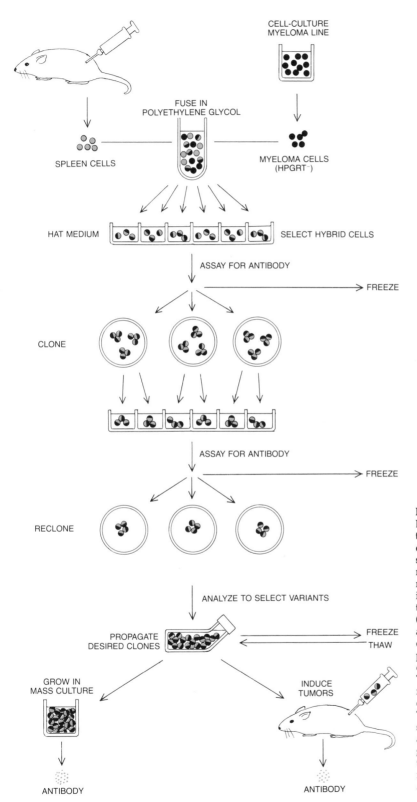

CELL-CULTURE
MYELOMA LINE

FUSE IN
POLYETHYLENE GLYCOL

SPLEEN CELLS

MYELOMA CELLS
(HPGRT⁻)

HAT MEDIUM — SELECT HYBRID CELLS

ASSAY FOR ANTIBODY

→ FREEZE

CLONE

ASSAY FOR ANTIBODY

→ FREEZE

RECLONE

ANALYZE TO SELECT VARIANTS

PROPAGATE
DESIRED CLONES

→ FREEZE
← THAW

GROW IN
MASS CULTURE

INDUCE
TUMORS

ANTIBODY

ANTIBODY

Figure 10.3 STANDARD PROCE-DURE for deriving monoclonal antibodies begins with the fusion, mediated by polyethylene glycol, of spleen cells from an immunized mouse (or rat) with mouse (or rat) myeloma cells. Hybrids are selected in a medium containing hypoxanthine, aminopterin, and thymidine (HAT). The medium is assayed for antibody secretion, and a portion of each positive culture is frozen as a precaution. Positive cultures are cloned and the clones are assayed. The positive ones are then frozen, recloned and assayed for the presence of immunoglobulin variants. The clones finally selected can be stored frozen. When the samples are thawed, they can be either grown in culture to produce the antibody or injected into animals to induce myelomas that secrete the antibody.

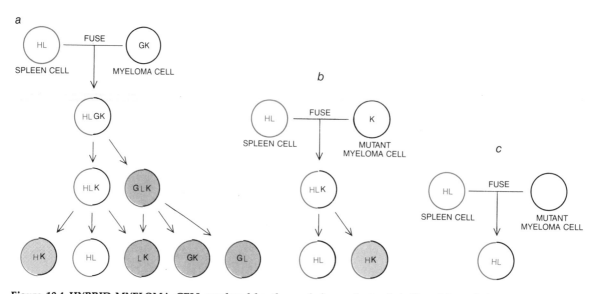

Figure 10.4 HYBRID-MYELOMA CELL produced by the usual fusion process (*a*) synthesizes not only the heavy (*H*) and light (*L*) chains of its spleen-cell parent but also the gamma (*G*) heavy and the kappa (*K*) light chains of its myeloma parent: it is thus designated HLGK. Hybrids tend to lose chromosomes, so that as the clone grows some chains are lost as is indicated here. Cultures are assayed to select desired variants (*unshaded cells*) until a stable HL variant secreting only specific antibody (or for some purposes an HK variant) is isolated. Fusion with mutant myeloma cells that make only a K chain (*b*) or no immunoglobulin at all (*c*) makes it easier to derive the desired HL clone.

range of substances: the small antigens called haptens; proteins (including enzymes), carbohydrates and glycolipids; cell-surface components and viruses. The methods seem to be generally applicable. If the animal makes a certain antibody, one should be able to immortalize the antibody as a hybrid myeloma. The degree of difficulty in deriving a specific hybrid myeloma seems to vary with the immune response of the animal. When the response is very weak, the search for a hybrid clone secreting the specific antibody among the many clones secreting nonspecific immunoglobulins can require special procedures. We have developed several ways of screening large numbers of cells or clones for antibody production; we have also learned how to preselect spleens that are enriched in cells producing the specific antibody. There are no miracles, however. If the animal does not make an antibody, there is no way to immortalize that antibody.

A monoclonal antibody is a well-defined chemical reagent that can be reproduced at will, in contrast to a conventional antiserum, which is a variable mixture of reagents and can never be reproduced once the original supply has been exhausted. As monoclonals become available they are therefore likely to supersede conventional antibodies in many investigative and clinical laboratories. An example is provided by the standard test for the blood groups *A*, *B*, *AB* and *O*. Reagents for the test (antibodies to the *A* and *B* red-cell antigens) are conventionally obtained from human serum. The best results are obtained by hyperimmunizing the donor of the serum by injecting red cells of the appropriate group (or better, a purified antigen), a potentially hazardous procedure; where such hyperimmunization is not done, as in the U.K., the reagents tend to be of lower quality. Moreover, the donated serum must be carefully screened for the presence of unwanted antibodies whose activity might obscure the anti-*A* or the anti-*B* reaction. (That is why reagents for the test cannot be obtained by immunizing laboratory animals. Antibodies in the animal serum would recognize the human character of the red cells being tested, completely eliminating the distinction between the *A* and the *B* groups.)

We have been able to establish that a monoclonal antibody to the individual specificity of a blood group need not be of human origin. In collaboration with Lennox, Steven Sacks and others a reagent is being produced at the Medical Research Council Laboratory of Molecular Biology from mass cultures of hybrid-myeloma cells that specifically recognizes Group *A* antigen. The reagent has been tested in comparison with the best available commercial reagents by Douglas Voak and Jack Darnborough of the Cambridge Regional Blood Transfusion Center and has been found to be equally effective.

The ability to derive antibodies to a single component of a "dirty" mixture opens up a new approach to the purification of natural products. As we became convinced of this premise we felt it needed to be put to the most stringent test we could think of. The substance of choice was interferon, which is notoriously difficult to purify and to obtain in significant quantity. When Secher and Derek C. Burke of the University of Warwick set out to purify interferon by immunoadsorption, the best interferon preparations to which they had access were about 1 percent pure. They immunized mice with a prepa-

ration of this crude interferon, fused spleen cells from the immunized mice with mouse myeloma cells and then tested the hybrid clones for their production of anti-interferon antibody, supplementing the unreliable and laborious biological assay for anti-interferon activity with tests for immunoglobulin secretion. With much difficulty they were able to select a positive clone, and by injecting its cells into mice they induced tumors that secreted the antibody in large amounts. The antibody was attached to carbohydrate beads to prepare an immunoadsorbent column. Passing a totally crude interferon preparation through the column purified it 5,000-fold in a single step. Purification on an industrial scale is now being explored (see Figure 10.5).

Monoclonal antibodies can be prepared that are specific for individual components of any complex mixture, and unlimited amounts of each antibody can be produced for immunoadsorbent columns. This makes it possible to dissect a mixture of completely unknown substances into its components.

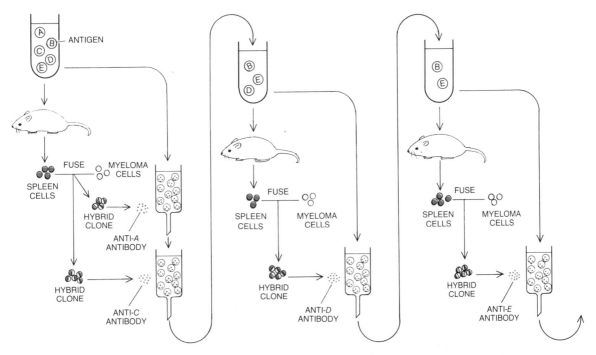

Figure 10.5 UNKNOWN MIXTURE can in effect be dissected by the monoclonal antibodies it engenders. A random set of antibodies, derived by immunizing animals with the unknown mixture, are applied to immunoadsorbent columns, which remove the corresponding antigens. The depleted mixture, now enriched in the remaining antigens, is injected to produce more antibody, and so on in cascade fashion. Hybrid-myeloma cells therefore provide a tool for characterizing the components and at the same time for separating and purifying them.

Animals are immunized with the mixture to be analyzed; hybrid-myeloma clones are derived and the antibodies from each clone serve to remove the components from the mixture one by one in cascade fashion.

One of the most exciting investigative applications of monoclonal antibodies is in the area of membrane biology. Membrane proteins are hard to purify. They are present in cells in small amounts; often they have no easily measured biological activity, or else their activity is destroyed when the membranes are solubilized for analysis. One way to overcome these problems is to characterize cell-surface molecules by immunological methods, an approach that has been fruitful in the recognition of surface antigens that characterize particular cell types at different stages of tissue differentiation. Conventional antibodies to surface antigens are usually complex, however, and do not recognize single molecules; elaborate procedures have been required to circumvent this complexity.

In 1977 Galfré and I, along with Alan F. Williams of the University of Oxford, showed how the hybrid-myeloma technique could identify individual differentiation antigens. We immunized a mouse with cell membranes from rat thymus. After immortalizing the mouse cells that secreted antibody to thymus lymphocytes we were able to isolate clones producing different specific antibodies. In that one attempt we defined three new antigenic specificities, a task that might have required years of sophisticated immunology by conventional methods. Since then a number of other monoclonal antibodies to differentiation antigens of mouse, rat and human cells have been prepared.

The antigenic structure of a cell's surface established the cell's lineage and defines subsets of cells. For example, B lymphocytes can be distinguished from T lymphocytes (which take part in cellular immune reactions rather than in the secretion of antibody) largely because the former have immunoglobulin molecules on their surface and the latter have characteristic markers such as the Thy-1 antigen. Most surface markers, however, are not specific for a single subset of cells. Even the B cell's characteristic immunoglobulin may be present in several functionally different members of the B-cell lineage, from the so-called memory cells (which respond to reimmunization with an antigen the organism has previously been exposed to) to plasma cells (which secrete antibody). What characterizes a particular differentiated state is the presence of a particular ensemble of surface antigens and their quantitative expression.

To establish a unique antigenic profile for each of many cell types will require a vast collection of monoclonal antibodies and will take a long time. A good start has been made with the few reagents already available and with the help of cytofluorometers and fluorescence-activated cell sorters: instruments that can quickly measure both the size and the fluorescent intensity of large numbers of cells to which monoclonal antibodies, tagged with a fluorescent dye, have been attached. A large cell population can thus be fractionated into subpopulations on the basis of their size and surface-antigen pattern, and then the function of each subpopulation can be studied. Monoclonal antibodies, in other words, are standard reagents that can identify new surface molecules and at the same time distinguish among cell populations. So far the best results have been reported with various blood-forming and lymphoid cells; one directly practical application has been the differential diagnosis of various leukemias and related disorders.

The pattern of reactivity of monoclonal antibodies against subpopulations of cells is sometimes consistent with a given cell line's pattern of maturation, but not always. One monoclonal antibody seems to recognize an antigen characteristic of certain bone-marrow cells in the rat, whereas in the peripheral lymphoid organs it recognizes lymphocytes and in nervous tissue it recognizes some component that is as yet unidentified. Among the peripheral lymphocytes the antigen is present on T cells but not on B cells; yet it reappears on plasma cells, which are derived from B cells. We say this monoclonal antibody recognizes a kind of "jumping" antigenic determinant.

The monoclonal approach to characterizing differentiation antigens thus makes it possible to probe for the particular stage at which an antigen is expressed as well as for the line of cells that expresses it. The cascade purification method I described above can be applied not only to characterize the antigenic complexity of the cell surface but also to dissect functional as well as structural components of other biological materials such as cell organelles and pharmacologically active cell extracts.

The "monospecificity" of antibodies from hybrid-myeloma clones has thrown new light on some well-known phenomena of antigen-antibody reactions. One indication of the binding of antigen to conventional antibodies in a test tube, for example, is the formation of a precipitate. The effect is not generally observed when the antibody is monoclonal. This is perhaps the first formal proof of the theory, advanced more than 40 years ago, that the precipitate is a three-dimensional lattice of antigens and antibodies. A monoclonal antibody binds only to a single antigenic determinant on an antibody molecule, so that no such lattice can be formed by a monoclonal antibody and most antigens. It can be formed only if the antigen is a polymer composed of repeated identical structural elements.

Monospecificity has also revealed some hitherto unsuspected phenomena that call for new interpretations of antigen-antibody reactions. To take just one example, it appears that the binding of different antibodies to neighboring sites on the same antigen is an important factor in the rupture of a cell membrane by complement. This synergistic effect was discovered as we were isolating the rat antibodies to histocompatibility antigens. We assayed for the presence of antibody-secreting hybrid myelomas by measuring the cytotoxic, or cell-killing, activity of their culture mediums. The supernatants of the uncloned cultures were consistently cytotoxic, but once we had cloned individual cells their supernatants showed no such activity. It occurred to Howard to measure the activity of a mixture of the supernatants of these apparently negative clones. To our delight the mixture was active, and then it was easy to purify two complementary components.

Once the synergistic effect was understood the "silent" activity of the isolated components could be exploited in a special way. Test cells could be "sensitized" by exposure to one monoclonal antibody and then exposed to the antibodies from other clones, thus revealing entire repertoires of antibodies that act synergistically. Clearly there are cases where mixtures of monoclonal antibodies will be essential to produce a desired effect. In each case a decision will have to be made whether the advantages of blending monoclonals in specific proportions (rather than relying on the uncontrollable mixtures present in ordinary antiserums) will justify the effort involved in deriving the monoclonals.

M onoclonal antibodies are slowly beginning to replace conventional antiserums in standard kits for such procedures as the radioimmunoassay; many commercial companies are marketing them. Because they can be produced in large quantities

they will make possible widespread use of kits of diagnostic reagents that until now were either not available at all or were considered too highly specialized for general application; one example is an antibody to the neurotransmitter called Substance P, derived recently by A. Claudio Cuello and me. The impact of monoclonals in virology, parasitology and bacteriology is only beginning to be felt. Great hopes are placed on their application to organ transplantation, just one aspect of which should be the worldwide standardization of tissue typing. In basic research the possibilities are even wider, with applications already reported in embryology and pharmacology and in the study of receptors for hormones and neurotransmitters.

Possible roles for monoclonal antibodies in direct therapy are under serious investigation. The most obvious role is in passive immunization (the injection of an antibody into a patient, as opposed to active immunization with an antigen that stimulates the patient's own antibody response). Given the impurity of conventional antibodies, passive immunization is not a common method of treatment, but it may prove to be effective when a purified antibody can be administered. In tumor therapy two kinds of roles are foreseen for monoclonal antibodies. One role is the targeting of toxic drugs: antibodies to the tissues of a particular organ or to specific tumor antigens could be attached to drug molecules to concentrate the drug's effect. Alternatively it may be possible to produce antitumor antibodies that will themselves find and attack tumor cells.

For therapeutic applications antibodies derived from human lymphocytes rather than from the mouse or the rat would be desirable. Contrary to early hopes, this has proved to be difficult; attempts to immortalize antibody-producing human cells by fusing them with mouse or rat myeloma cells have so far been disappointing. The problem is that when human cells are fused with animal cells, there is a rapid preferential loss of human chromosomes from the resulting interspecific hybrid cells. And so far the search for a suitable human myeloma line that can be cultured and fused to make an intraspecific hybrid has not borne fruit.

In this overview of the uses of hybrid-myeloma antibodies I have referred only superficially to their obvious applications in basic immunological research. I have preferred to emphasize the fact that, although the technique originated in our effort to understand the genetic organization and expression of immunoglobulins, there has already been an impressive "spin-off" into many other areas. It is always hard to define the boundary between basic and applied research, but to experience personally the transition from one to the other has made a deep impression on me. I cannot think that if my research aim five or six years ago had been the production of monoclonal antibodies, I would ever have stumbled on the idea of attempting simultaneously to derive mutant antibody-secreting cells in one corner of the laboratory and to fuse two myeloma cells in another corner. Yet that was the combination that led to the initial production of monoclonal antibodies against sheep red blood cells.

Catalytic Antibodies

This new class of molecules couples antibodies' vast diversity with the catalytic power that makes enzymes invaluable for technology, medicine and basic research.

• • •

Richard A. Lerner and Alfonso Tramontano
March, 1988

Can antibodies be made to serve as enzymes? These two classes of proteins seem to have evolved for different tasks. Enzymes are distinguished by their catalytic ability, the ability to accelerate chemical reactions without being used up themselves. Antibodies are unique in their ability to recognize a diversity of substances.

Yet both classes of proteins exert their effects in much the same way: by binding to other molecules. Enzymes have a cleft or crevice on their surface, in which they bind chemical reactants in the course of transforming them. Antibodies have a specialized site that enables them to bind to molecules belonging to foreign organisms that have invaded the body, thereby marking the intruders for destruction by other components of the immune system.

The great diversity of antibodies is a reflection of the immune system's defensive function. In its ability to make perhaps 100 million different antibodies, each one capable of binding to a particular foreign substance, the immune system in effect anticipates the multitude and variety of possible invaders. The chemical reactions of life, in contrast, are stereotyped and invariant. Nature is satisfied with perhaps a few thousand enzymes, each one capable of catalyzing one or a few reactions.

Without a catalyst most biochemical reactions proceed with impossible slowness. Whether they take place in living organisms, in the laboratory or in industrial processes, these transformations depend crucially on the small array of existing enzymes. Yet for a reaction that is not biologically essential there is often no enzyme. The immune system, however, can make an antibody to almost any substance, and it is now possible to isolate a supply of pure "monoclonal" antibody that has a single target molecule. Is there any way to build on the basic similarity between antibodies and enzymes in order to give antibodies the ability to catalyze chemical reactions?

In our laboratories at the Research Institute of Scripps Clinic we have been learning about the structural details of an antibody's interaction with its target molecule. Recently this new knowledge, combined with other chemical intuitions, has suggested ways to harness for catalysis the energy with which antibodies bind to their targets. We have already produced the first catalytic antibodies, and the research could ultimately bear fruit in a virtually limitless variety of catalytic antibodies for use in biotechnology, medicine and investigations of protein structure and function.

Even though ordinary antibodies do not catalyze reactions in living organisms, they do show certain features suggesting a potential for catalysis. Working with Elizabeth D. Getzoff and John A. Tainer of Scripps and H. Mario Geysen of the Commonwealth Serum Laboratories in Australia, we found that antibodies can induce structural changes in their target molecules. We first elicited antibodies to a protein by injecting it into experimental animals. We went on to determine which parts of the original protein the resulting antibodies bound to most readily and how they gained access to those antigenic segments.

As a prototypical target protein we chose myohemerythrin (MHR), which serves in certain marine worms as an oxygen carrier. Like other proteins, MHR consists of a long chain of amino acids, folded into a specific three-dimensional form. The sequence of MHR's amino acids is known, and its three-dimensional fold was determined through X-ray crystallography by Steven Sheriff of the National Institute of Diabetes and Digestive and Kidney Diseases, Wayne A. Hendrickson of Columbia University and Janet D. Smith of Purdue University. The sequence information enabled us to synthesize peptides—short sequences of amino acids—mimicking segments of the protein. The structural information then told us which site on the protein each of the peptides represented (see Figure 11.1).

We tested each peptide for its ability to interact with anti-MHR antibodies and took the result as a measure of antibody binding to the corresponding site on the folded protein. The resulting antigenic map of MHR showed that every site on the protein is the target of a few antibodies, but the most reactive sites are those at which the protein's structure is flexible and its amino acids form a convex surface, which presumably fits the concave binding pocket of one or another antibody.

We then examined the antibodies' binding preferences in more detail. To find out which amino acids are crucial to binding at a given site, we synthesized peptides mimicking the antigenic site at every amino acid but one, where a different amino acid was substituted. Again we tested the peptides for their reactivity with anti-MHR antibodies, noting the effect of each substitution. If a substitution reduced the reactivity substantially, the original amino acid must be involved in antibody binding.

To our surprise, not all the amino acids crucial to binding can be found on the surface of the protein, where they are directly exposed to antibodies. In one sequence of amino acids representing an antigenic site, for example, antibodies must interact with the amino acids valine, tyrosine and glutamic acid to bind effectively. Replacing any one of the three sharply reduces the reactivity of the peptide. Now, the three-dimensional structure of MHR shows that only valine and glutamic acid are available at the surface of the protein; tyrosine (and in particular its bulky side chain) is buried in the protein's interior. It is hidden under the glutamic acid and another nearby amino acid, lysine, which are held together by a weak electrostatic bond. The tyrosine residue would seem to be inaccessible to an antibody interacting with the surface of MHR.

As the antibody binds, then, the tyrosine must somehow be presented on the protein surface. If the structure in which tyrosine is buried is the protein's stablest (lowest-energy) configuration, then the bound antibody must hold the protein in a relatively high-energy form. The antibody must expend energy to do so; the source of the energy must be the antibody's binding strength.

Proteins are dynamic molecules; their bonds forever stretch, twist and vibrate. It may be that the tyrosine side chain occasionally rotates out to the surface of the protein, breaking the weak bond between glutamic acid and lysine, and is stabilized there by the bound antibody (see Figure 11.2). Alternatively, the initial interactions of the antibody with the protein may foster the cleavage of the bond. The buried side chain could then rotate outward to interact directly with the antibody.

In either case, the results say something of fundamental importance about antibodies and their binding ability: some antibodies may bind most readily to high-energy states of their target molecules. In stabilizing these states the antibodies in effect overcome bonds or forces that exist in the targets' low-energy form. In this, antibodies are something like enzymes. Enzymes also alter bonds in their substrates, or target molecules. To be sure, the covalent bonds broken by enzymes are much stronger than the ones overcome by antibodies. Yet enzymes bind to their targets no more strongly, on the whole, than antibodies do. If binding energy is responsible for the catalytic ability of enzymes, might antibody binding also be put to work so that instead of simply labeling their targets, antibodies actually transformed them chemically?

The way enzymes work suggests a means of doing just that. The effect of an enzyme can be

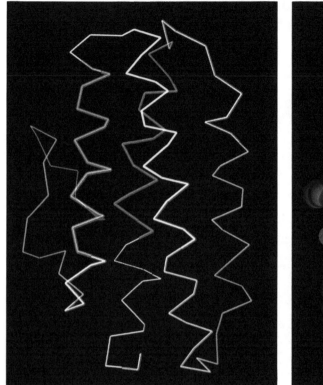 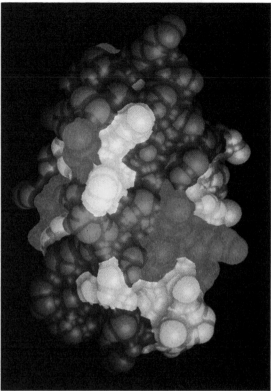

Figure 11.1 MYOHEMERYTHRIN (MHR), the oxygen-carrying protein of a marine worm, was mapped to show antibodies' binding preferences. Peptide molecules mimicking short segments in the protein chain (*left*) where synthesized. The degree to which antibodies elicited by the whole protein reacted with each peptide was mapped onto the protein surface (*right*). The most reactive regions are red, regions of intermediate reactivity are yellow and the lest reactive regions are blue. The antibodies preferred sites at which the surface is convex and the protein's chemical groups are highly mobile. Both traits may ensure a good fit between the binding pocket and the surface.

understood in terms of the energetic demands of a reaction (see Figure 11.3). Chemical processes can be described by energy surfaces in which stable molecules are defined by deep wells. For one molecule to be transformed into another, its atoms must travel across the energy surface from one well to another. The atoms must first gain energy until they reach a crest and then lose energy to fall into the stable product well. The highest point on the reaction path correspond to a dynamic, unstable transition state in which bonds are only partially formed or broken. The transition state exists for just a fleeting instant during the journey from reactants to products.

The difference in height of the points on the energy surface representing the starting materials and the transition state is the reaction's activation energy. It is the energy barrier that must be surmounted before the reaction can coast to completion. The higher a reaction's activation energy is, the slower it proceeds. An enzyme speeds up a reaction by lowering its activation energy: changing the topography of the energy surface to provide a pathway crossing a smaller energy "hill."

In 1946 Linus Pauling suggested one way in which an enzyme might lower a reaction's energy barrier: by binding most strongly not to the reactants but to the transition state. The transition state is thereby stabilized, and as a result less energy is needed to form it; the reaction is accelerated, often

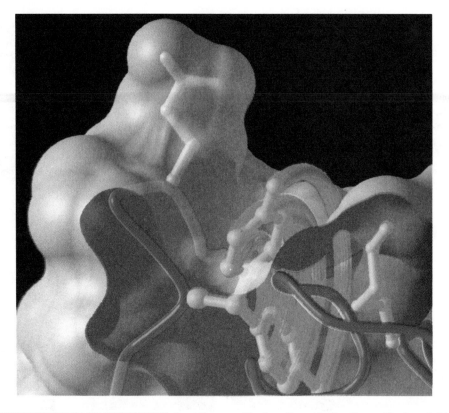

Figure 11.2 TYROSINE SIDE CHAIN ROTATES about the protein backbone (*red*) when an antibody binds to the antigenic site. The rearrangement may occur through random thermal motion and simply be stabilized by the bound antibody; alternatively, the antibody might actively reshape the surface of the protein and induce the change in amino acid conformation.

Figure 11.3 ENERGY PROFILE charts the energetic demands of a hypothetical chemical reaction, from reactants to products. From its starting point the curve rises by an amount representing the reaction's activation energy. It reaches a peak corresponding to the reaction's transition state, an ephemeral complex of atoms that has no resting state. Enzymes catalyze a reaction in part by binding to the transition state and thereby stabilizing it. The activation energy of the uncatalyzed reaction (*black curve*) is lowered (*colored curve*) and the process is accelerated, often by a factor of several billion.

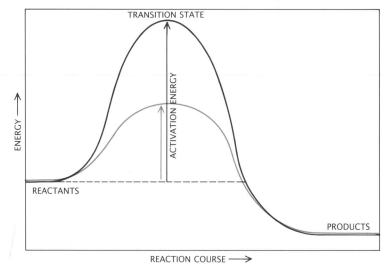

by factors of several billion. The enzyme's effect is catalytic because the products diffuse away from it, enabling it to bind and transform molecules of the substrate repeatedly.

In Pauling's scheme the fundamental difference between the actions of enzymes and antibodies is that whereas enzymes bind most readily to high-energy activated states, antibodies bind to low-energy structures. Many years ago William P. Jencks of Brandeis University proposed that if one could develop an antibody to a transition state (a high-energy structure), that antibody might have a catalytic effect on the corresponding chemical reaction.

An effort to develop antibodies that bind to a transition state faces a practical problem, however. To elicit antibodies one needs an antigen, which is injected into an experimental animal to induce an immune response. Here the true antigen is unavailable: the transition state itself is so unstable that for practical purposes it does not exist. An answer to the dilemma came from another of Pauling's proposals. He predicted that, given a reaction for which an enzyme exists, a stable substance might mimic the transition state in shape and charge. Such a transition-state analogue would bind very tightly to the enzyme, inhibiting its catalytic action by filling the binding pocket and preventing it from binding to its true substrate. Over the past 20 years a number of compounds have been synthesized that behave the way Pauling predicted.

Such a transition-state analogue, then, might serve as an antigen that would induce antibodies capable of recognizing the actual transition state, stabilizing it and perhaps acting on the substrate as a true catalyst. We began our exploration of the possibility by focusing on a reaction known as ester hydrolysis, in which a water molecule attacks a chemical group known as an ester to produce a molecule of an acid and a molecule of an alcohol (see Figure 11.4). An ester group consists of a central carbon atom bound to two oxygen atoms and another carbon. The central carbon is doubly bonded to one of the oxygens, with which it forms the acid product; the other oxygen, which is destined to become part of the alcohol product, links up with another organic group. In the hydrolysis reaction the bond between the central carbon and the oxygen of the alcohol group is broken and a new bond forms between the carbon and the oxygen in water.

The four atoms of the ester bear little charge and

lie in a plane. As a water molecule interacts with the ester, however, the reaction passes through a transition state in which the central carbon is surrounded by a tetrahedral arrangement of three oxygens, some of them carrying an electric charge, and a carbon. In the transition state the bonds not only are reoriented but also are stretched to perhaps 120 percent of their normal length. The distinctive features of the transition state indicate that the ester itself cannot serve as an antigen for inducing catalytic antibodies. The ester would elicit antibodies capable of recognizing and stabilizing only the starting material of the reaction. Such antibodies would increase rather than lower the reaction's energy barrier.

What is needed is a transition-state analogue. Substituting a phosphorus for the central carbon in the transition state's tetrahedral ensemble of atoms yields a stable compound known as a phosphonate ester. The distribution of charge on the oxygen atoms of the molecule resembles that of the transition state. In addition the phosphorus-oxygen bonds are about 20 percent longer than ordinary carbon-oxygen bonds, which enables the analogue to mimic the elongated bonds of the transition state.

We synthesized such an analogue, coupled it to a carrier protein and immunized mice with the conjugate. We then extracted antibody-secreting spleen cells from the mice. We fused the spleen cells with tumor cells to generate clones of identical antibody-secreting cells. An antigen ordinarily induces the production of many different antibodies that bind to many different sites on the molecule, but each antibody-secreting cell (and the clone derived from it) makes just one kind of antibody. In order to find cells that were secreting antibody to the transition-state analogue and not, say, to sites on the carrier protein, we tested each monoclonal antibody for the ability to bind to the transition-state analogue.

Having identified monoclonal antibodies specific for the analogue, we tested their ability to catalyze the hydrolysis of the corresponding ester. Some of the antibodies had no effect; perhaps they were specific for a feature of the molecule that is not matched in the transition state itself. But we were gratified to find that other antibodies actually behaved as catalysts and accelerated the ester hydrolysis by a factor of about 1,000. As we expected, the phosphonate ester with which the antibodies had been induced inhibited their catalytic action, presumably by preempting the binding of the substrate. Like the recognition ability of ordinary anti-

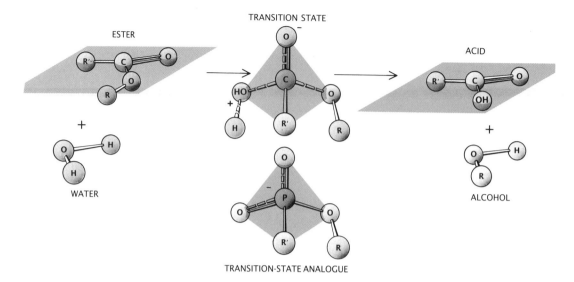

Figure 11.4 HYDROLOSIS OF AN ESTER passes through an unstable transition state whose distinctive shape and charge can be mimicked by a stable molecule. The ester group and the acid product, which inherits the ester's central carbon, have a planar geometry and carry no electric charge (R and R' represent chemical groups that do not take part in the reaction.) The transition state is tetrahedral and is polarized: a partial negative charge is concentrated at one apex. A stable analogue, in which phosphorus takes the place of the central carbon in the transition state, mimics its geometry and approximates its distribution of charge.

bodies, the catalytic activity of these molecules was highly specific: they catalyzed hydrolysis only for esters having a transition-state structure that closely matched the immunizing antigen.

At about the same time as we did our experiments Scott J. Pollack, Jeffrey W. Jacobs and Peter G. Schultz of the University of California at Berkeley carried out a somewhat different experiment based on the same principle. They began with an antibody specific for phosphoryl choline, a molecule containing a phosphorus atom tetrahedrally bound to four oxygens. The three-dimensional structure of the antibody had been solved by David R. Davies and his colleagues at the National Institute of Arthritis, Metabolism, and Digestive Diseases, and it suggested that the binding pocket neatly accommodated the tetrahedral phosphate group.

The Berkeley team reasoned that this antibody might stabilize the transition state for a hydrolysis reaction and thereby catalyze the process. The group therefore set about designing a reactant that would give rise to a transition state resembling phosphoryl choline in charge and shape. To pass through a tetrahedral transition state containing four oxygens, the reactant had to contain a carbon-

ate group (a carbon coupled to three oxygens). When the investigators synthesized an appropriate carbonate, they found that their antibody accelerated its hydrolysis many hundredfold.

The Berkeley result supports the concept that stabilizing the transition state is the key to catalysis by antibodies. To demonstrate the broader principle, that it is possible to extract a catalyst of predetermined specificity from the immune system, one has to begin as we did, with an antigen. Our experiment points to a general scheme for developing catalytic antibodies. From study of chemical mechanisms one infers the shape and charge distribution of a reaction's transition state. Basic chemical considerations guide the design of a stable transition-state mimic, which serves to elicit an antibody with a complementary binding pocket. The development of catalytic antibodies, then, is largely a matter of designing and preparing the proper antigen.

The catalytic antibodies produced by careful antigen design can show not only chemical selectivity and catalytic efficiency but also a third property characteristic of enzymes: the ability to distinguish between stereochemically different forms of a molecule. In particular, molecules that contain a carbon atom bound to four different groups can exist in two forms that are chemically identical but are mirror images, related to each other as the left and right hands are related. The two enantiomers, or mirror-image forms, of such a chiral compound react identically with other, nonchiral substances. In a reaction between two chiral compounds, however, specific enantiomers may interact preferentially, just as there is a specific match between each hand and its respective glove.

All but one of the amino acids are chiral, and so are the proteins they compose. Most living things build their proteins from only one enantiomer of each amino acid. Hence enzymes, like other proteins, exist in only one chiral form. In a reaction that has a chiral starting material or product, an enzyme often will selectively catalyze the process for only one enantiomer. One would expect catalytic antibodies—which are chiral proteins themselves—to show the same stereospecificity.

Working with Andrew Napper and Stephen J. Benkovic of Pennsylvania State University, we tested for stereospecificity by studying a reaction in which the substrate, transition state and product are all chiral (see Figure 11.5). The reaction forms a bond between an oxygen at one end of a chainlike molecule and a carbon at the other end, transforming the starting material into a ring molecule called a lactone. A carbon atom in the middle of the chain is bound to four different groups and is chiral. It defines two enantiomers of the substrate, the transition state and the products. A stereospecific catalyst should preferentially bind to one enantiomer of the transition state, thereby transforming just one form of the substrate into one form of the product.

The reaction passes through a tetrahedral transition state resembling the transition state for ester hydrolysis. As before, we created a transition-state analogue by replacing the tetrahedral carbon with a phosphorus atom. We injected the analogue into experimental animals and obtained monoclonal antibodies. Although the analogue was a mixture of chiral forms, each monoclonal antibody recognized only one enantiomer. One of these antibodies had a catalytic effect. As expected, the catalyzed reaction

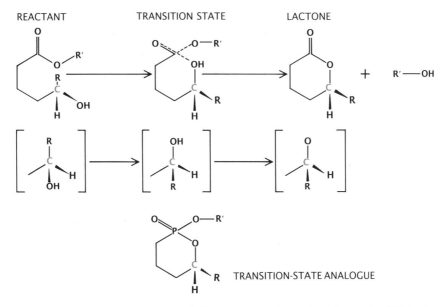

Figure 11.5 TEST OF STEREOSPECIFICITY for catalytic antibodies was a reaction in which a molecule containing an open chain of oxygen and carbon atoms is transformed into a lactone. The starting material, the transition state and the product all contain a chiral carbon (*color*): a carbon bound to four chemical groups that can have two mirror-image configurations (*top and middle*). The authors synthesized a transition-state analogue and made an antibody that would bind to just one form of the analogue. The antibody catalyzed the formation of only one form of lactone, which shows it was stereospecific: it distinguished between the chiral forms of the transition state.

consumed only half of the starting material, in which enantiomers of the progenitor molecule were mixed, and it yielded just one chiral form of the lactone product. The antibody's action, then, was stereospecific, presumably because its binding pocket was shaped to recognize only one form of the reaction's transition state.

Stereospecificity is likely to be a general property of catalytic antibodies, and it could suit them to a role in a number of industrial processes, including the synthesis of therapeutic drugs. Certain drug molecules contain one or more chiral centers, which give rise to several stereochemically different forms of the drug. Usually only one form of the molecule reacts properly with the drug's receptor site in the target cell. The wrong form can be useless or, if it reacts with unintended receptors in the body, even harmful.

The same considerations that enabled us to produce catalytic antibodies for reactions of simple molecules such as esters point the way to making antibodies for cleaving proteins and nucleic acids — the fundamental molecules of life and hence the principal materials of molecular biology and biotechnology. The structural bonds in proteins are amide bonds, which join a carbon in one amino acid to a nitrogen in an adjacent amino acid on the protein chain. In the transition state for amide hydrolysis the carbon at one end of the bond adopts a tetrahedral geometry much like the transition state in ester hydrolysis — a configuration readily mimicked with a phosphorus-containing analogue. An antibody elicited with such an analogue, which might also include a few of the amino acids flanking the target bond on the protein chain, might cleave a protein. Its action would be highly specific: it would hydrolyze only the bond residing within the amino acid sequence mimicked by the analogue.

Amide bonds are exceedingly stable, however, and antibodies capable of accelerating their hydrolysis have yet to be devised. One difficulty may be that simple transition-state binding is not enough for accelerating reactions whose activation energy is very high. The binding pocket of the catalytic protein (whether it is an antibody or an enzyme) must also be able to intervene directly in the reaction, changing its chemical mechanism so that a molecule is able to cross the energy surface from the substrate well to the product well by an alternative pathway of lower energy. That is, the amino acids lining the binding pocket must take part directly in the reaction.

The action of the amino acids (or, more precisely, their side chains) is analogous to the catalytic effect of simple compounds or ions in solution. Unlike enzymes, these species are too small to enclose the substrate in a binding pocket, and yet they can act as catalysts by forming transient chemical bonds with the reacting atoms. A simple base, for example, can accelerate ester hydrolysis by removing a hydrogen ion from a water molecule. The resulting hydroxide ion reacts with the ester group much more readily than the water molecule does on its own. Alternatively, a small molecule with an affinity for carbon can substitute for the water molecule to break the carbon-oxygen bond, releasing the alcohol and forming a complex, or intermediate, with the remainder of the ester. A water molecule then displaces the catalyst and releases the acid product of the hydrolysis.

The amino acid side chains in an enzyme's binding pocket have an advantage over catalytic groups in free solution in that they need not rely on chance to bring them together with the target molecule. In many enzymes three or more groups interact simultaneously with the substrate. If those groups existed as small molecules in a solution, their juxtaposition would be quite unlikely, even disregarding the requirement that they all be oriented properly. By aligning active groups with one another and with the bound substrate, the binding pocket of the enzyme makes possible catalytic mechanisms that would be virtually ruled out otherwise.

For example, the "catalytic triad" of the amino acids aspartate, histidine and serine, precisely positioned within the enzyme binding pocket, is known to be crucial to the functioning of trypsin and other enzymes that break down proteins in the digestive tract (see Figure 11.6). As the enzyme attacks an amide bond the three amino acids act in unison to dismantle the bond, step by step. First the carbon at one end of the amide bond is linked to the serine and the part of the protein ending with the nitrogen is released; then a water molecule reacts with the serine-substrate complex to release the remainder of the protein and restore the enzyme to its resting state (see Figure 11.7).

Hence, by direct participation of side chains in the binding pocket, an enzyme can break down a reaction that ordinarily passes through one high-energy transition state into a series of simple steps having

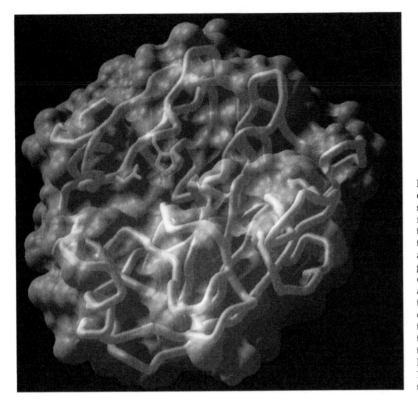

Figure 11.6 TRYPSIN, a digestive enzyme that catalyzes the hydrolysis of proteins, speeds the reaction not only by stabilizing the transition state as an amide (carbon-nitrogen) bond is broken but also by acting chemically on the amide group, through amino acid side chains in the binding pocket. Three amino acids (*green*) form a "catalytic triad" in trypsin and several related enzymes. The side chains react with the bound protein to form transition states of lower energy than the transition state of the uncatalyzed hydrolysis reaction (see Figure 11.7). The image shows the protein's surface and backbone.

transition states of lower energy. It is convenient to describe this aspect of enzyme action as a process distinct from transition-state binding, but in fact the two functions are linked. The binding pocket of the enzyme may stabilize the subsidiary transition states, lowering the energetic cost of their formation, as well as taking part in them directly through amino acid side chains.

In antibodies too the binding pocket is lined with precisely oriented side chains, some of which could well play a role in catalysis. Can the immune system be coaxed into producing an antibody whose binding pocket not only would stabilize a reaction's transition state but also would take part in the reaction directly and alter its pathway? Antibody molecules have their greatest variability in the segments of protein making up their binding pockets; even antibodies that recognize the same antigen may have pockets containing different sets of amino acids. Through meticulous antigen design it might be possible to elicit an antibody bearing specific amino acids that could participate in a reaction. One might, for example, try to design not a static mimic of the transition state but a dynamic one: a compound that, in imitation of the transition state, would react chemically with the binding pocket of an appropriate antibody.

Indeed, the staggering variability of antibody binding sites opens the possibility of developing antibodies that would bring many different sets of catalytic side chains to bear on the same reaction. Each of hundreds or thousands of antibodies to the same transition-state analogue might catalyze the reaction by a slightly different mechanism, depending on the constellation of side chains in the binding pocket. We have already seen some evidence for a diversity of mechanisms in our catalytic antibodies for ester hydrolysis: whereas our first antibody accelerates the reaction by a factor of 1,000, other antibodies to the same transition-state analogue accelerate the reaction by a factor of as much as seven million.

Such a diversity of catalytic mechanisms could

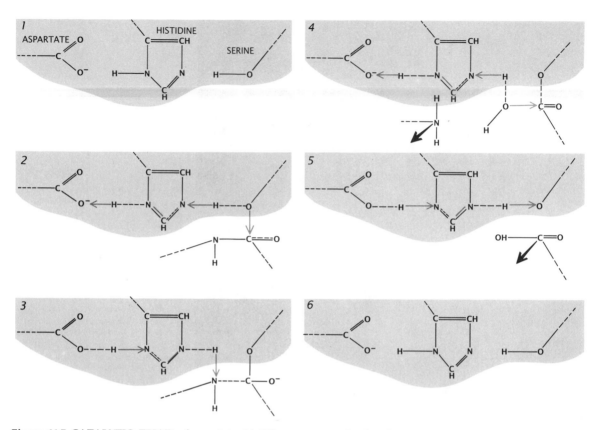

Figure 11.7 CATALYTIC TRIAD of aspartate, histidine and serine (*1*) acts in concert to break an amide bond of a protein in the active site of trypsin. The oxygen on serine is freed to attack the carbon as a proton (a hydrogen ion) is attracted from histidine to the negatively charged oxygen of aspartate, and another proton shuttles from serine to histidine (*2*). The first proton then returns and the second one attacks the nitrogen (*3*). As part of the protein is released, a water molecule takes its place, and the proton shuttle is played out again, this time forming a hydroxide group (OH) that attacks the bond between the carbon and the oxygen on serine (*4*). The bond is broken, the remainder of the protein is released (*5*) and the catalytic triad is restored to its resting condition (*6*).

prove a boon for the study of protein catalysis. What specific features account for the remarkable efficiency of the enzymes found in nature? What features represent a minimum requirement for their activity? How might less efficient, evolutionarily more primitive enzymes have been structured? These questions have motivated detailed studies of existing enzymes. Study of the catalytic effect of antibodies whose binding pockets vary subtly in their makeup will provide an efficient new means of addressing such questions.

The catalytic antibodies devised so far by us and by others transform comparatively simple compounds. Much of the potential of these new protein catalysts for biotechnology and medicine depends on the development of antibodies that are able to act on proteins or nucleic acids. Existing proteases (protein-cleaving enzymes) are few in number and relatively nonspecific in their action: they cleave their target bond with little regard for its chemical surroundings. Catalytic antibodies might hydrolyze amide bonds that are resistant to the known proteases, and they might be much more sensitive to the specific amino acids flanking the target bond.

Such catalysts could be put to use in medicine — for example in vaccination. Current vaccines mimic a pathogen, such as a virus, in order to induce protective antibodies. An antiviral vaccine of the future might mimic just the transition state in the hydrolysis of one viral protein. It might induce catalytic antibodies that would protect the recipient by actively breaking down the invading virus. At the same time the antibodies would spare the host's own proteins. By the same principles one might stimulate the immune system of a patient with heart disease to produce antibodies that would break up the proteins in blood clots, forestalling heart attacks.

Catalytic antibodies, then, could extend the immune system's innate capacity to defend the body. They will certainly contribute to biotechnology and to basic research both in chemistry and in molecular biology. Those disciplines should profit directly, from an expanded molecular toolbox. They might also profit in unforeseen ways, from the opportunity to explore the full potential of protein binding pockets for fostering chemical reactions.

Immunotoxins

The idea is to link a toxic agent to a monoclonal antibody binding to a particular tumor antigen, thus fashioning a "magic bullet" that will destroy targeted cancer cells but leave normal cells unharmed

• • •

R. John Collier and Donald A. Kaplan
July, 1984

How is it possible to destroy a particular subset of a patient's own cells and leave the rest of the cells unaffected? This is the difficult objective in the chemotherapy of cancer and certain other diseases. A cancer cell is a normal cell gone wrong. Freed from the usual constraints on growth, it multiplies rapidly; the cancer invades adjacent tissue and may metastasize to distant tissues. Most of the chemotherapeutic agents now available to the oncologist are drugs that are taken up by, or that primarily affect, cells that are multiplying rapidly. Unfortunately, this is a marginal basis for selectivity. Normal cells are not unaffected by these drugs. Doses large enough to eradicate cancer cells with high efficiency can be lethal to the patient, and even moderate doses can cause a variety of harmful side effects.

There is an alternative approach: a "magic bullet" that destroys its designated targets without significantly affecting any other cells. Antibiotics are one kind of magic bullet. An antibiotic can kill bacteria or prevent their proliferation without harming human cells because it inhibits metabolic processes peculiar to the prokaryotic bacterial cell. It is harder to develop comparable selectively toxic

agents for fungal or parasitic diseases because the metabolism of the eukaryotic cells that cause them is too much like that of the infected mammalian host's cells.

A different kind of magic bullet would be one whose magic resides in its ability to home on a designated target such as a particular kind of cancer cell. That is, the toxic agent itself would be toxic for most cells, but it is allowed to reach only a defined population of cells. Within the past decade advances in cell-surface immunology, the advent of monoclonal antibodies and new understanding of certain highly toxic natural substances have begun to make such an approach seem feasible. The strategy is simple, at least in principle: Develop a monoclonal antibody that binds specifically to a target cell and not to other cells, and a couple the antibody to a toxic molecule. The antibody-toxin conjugate, or immunotoxin, should kill target cells, and no other cells, with high efficiency. In practice, as we shall explain, there are difficulties in this approach, and there is a long way to go before immunotoxins can become standard therapeutic agents. A number of investigators, however, have been able to demonstrate the capacity of immunotoxins for targeted killing of cells growing in a laboratory culture, and the method is being tested in animals.

The lipid surface membrane of a living cell is studded with hundreds of chemical structures (mostly proteins, some of them with carbohydrate chains attached) that have various roles in cell communication and metabolism. Many of the structures differ from species to species and from individual to individual of the same species; in an individual many of them differ from one cell type to another. Significantly, some cell-surface structures are peculiar to certain malignant cells, and they distinguish tumor cells even from normal cells of the same tissue.

When human cells are introduced into the body of an animal, cell-surface markers that are different from the recipient's own are recognized as being foreign. They therefore serve as antigens, and the animal's immune system responds to their presence by making antibodies against them. Antibodies are highly specific protein molecules that are able to recognize and bind tightly to the particular antigens that induced their synthesis. The natural function of such antibodies is to initiate the defensive processes that inactivate or destroy harmful foreign substances, but for some time investigators have exploited the specificity of antibodies to find, identify, label and separate particular cells or molecules. Antibodies elicited by particular human cells should therefore provide a means of distinguishing those cells from others. Indeed, early in this century the German bacteriologist and immunologist Paul Ehrlich proposed that antibodies might somehow serve to deliver chemically coupled toxic agents to particular cells.

For many years that was not possible. Until recently antibodies reacting specifically with only a single antigen, and therefore binding dependably to a single class of cells, could be obtained only in minute quantities because it was difficult to purify them from the mixture of antibodies in the serum of an immunized animal. Each specific antibody is synthesized and secreted by plasma cells derived from a particular clone of B lymphocytes dedicated to the synthesis of that antibody, but there was no way to propagate such a clone in the laboratory because the antibody-secreting cells could not be grown in a laboratory culture medium.

That problem was overcome by the development of hybridoma technology in 1975 by Cesar Milstein of the Medical Research Council Laboratory of Molecular Biology in Cambridge. Milstein found a way to fuse B lymphocytes with the related but malignant myeloma cells. The resulting hybridoma cells are like B cells in that each produces a single antibody; they are like myeloma cells in that they can be grown indefinitely in culture. A single hybridoma cell can be grown into a clone of identical cells, which serves as a continuing source of a "monoclonal" antibody against a specific antigen (see Figure 12.1).

To isolate a monoclonal antibody recognizing a certain type of cell one inoculates laboratory mice with a pure culture of the cells of interest or with a preparation of their cell membrane (which carries the cell-surface antigens). The animal's B cells are isolated and then fused with myeloma cells, and the resulting hybridomas are screened for the production of monoclonal antibodies that bind to the target cells in culture or to their membranes but do not bind effectively to a panel of control cells or membranes. The specificity of binding of monoclonal antibodies is rarely absolute, but it can be extremely high, in part because the antigen recognized by the antibody is much more prevalent on the surface of the target cells than it is on the surface of nontarget cells.

Even before monoclonal antibodies against cell-surface antigens became available, investigators had been studying the properties of toxic agents that might be delivered by antibodies to kill cancer cells. There are several candidates. There are toxic drugs, such as the ones we alluded to above that are currently administered for the chemotherapy of cancer. There are radioactive isotopes of various elements, some of which have an affinity for particular tissues (as iodine has for the thyroid gland). And there are naturally occurring toxic proteins produced by certain bacteria, plants and animals (see Figure 12.2).

All these candidates have been coupled to antibodies and tested, but most of the work on immunotoxins has been done with naturally occurring toxic proteins, some of which are among the most potent cytocidal (cell-killing) substances known. Under appropriate conditions a human cell can be killed by a single molecule of the toxin secreted by *Corynebacterium diphtheriae*, the agent that causes diphtheria, or of the protein ricin, which is found in castor beans. We have worked mainly with diphtheria toxin.

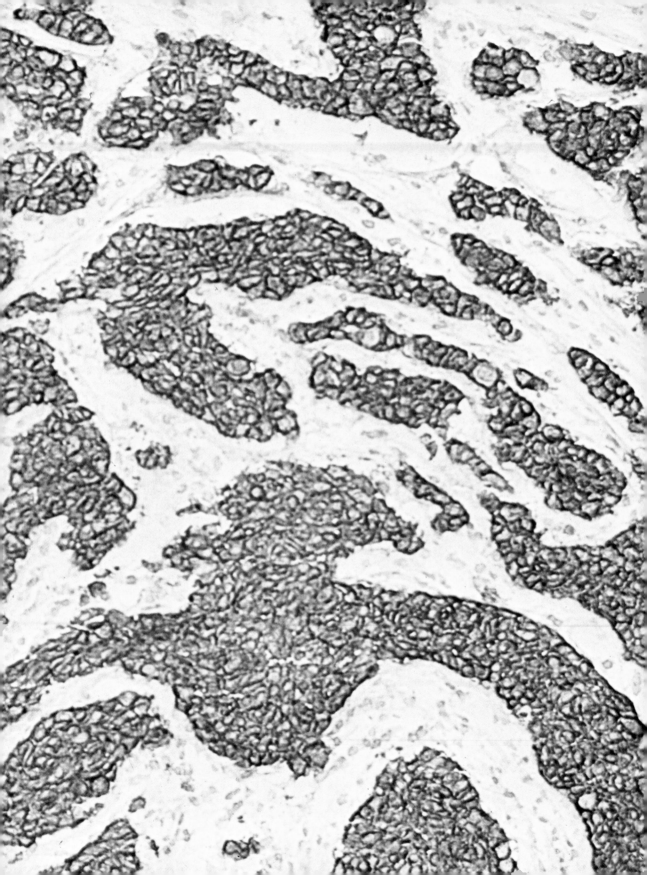

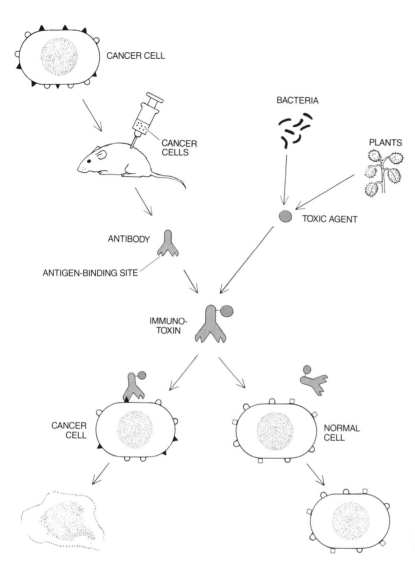

CANCER CELL

BACTERIA

PLANTS

CANCER CELLS

TOXIC AGENT

ANTIBODY

ANTIGEN-BINDING SITE

IMMUNO-TOXIN

CANCER CELL

NORMAL CELL

Figure 12.2 CONCEPT OF AN IMMUNOTOXIN is simple. Cancer cells, which include among their surface molecules a tumor-associated antigen (*black*), are injected into a mouse. The mouse synthesizes antibodies against the antigen. A toxic substance derived from a bacterial or other source is linked to the antibody to make an immunotoxin. The immunotoxin binds to the tumor-associated antigen on the cancer cells and kills the cells (*bottom left*). It does not bind to antigens on normal cells (*bottom right*), and so normal cells are not affected by the toxin.

Figure 12.1 MONOCLONAL ANTIBODIES home in on cancer cells in a frozen section taken from a breast carcinoma. The antibodies bind specifically to a tumor-associated antigen, a cell-surface molecule peculiar to the cancer cells. The antibodies are made visible by the indirect immunoperoxidase technique, by which the antibody-covered surface of each cancer is stained brown; the nuclei of both cancer cells and normal cells are counterstained light blue. Monoclonal antibodies such as the ones illustrated here are linked to toxic agents to make immunotoxins: composite molecules that bind to cancer cells and kill them but fail to bind to normal cells, leaving them unaffected.

The toxin is an enzyme that inactivates an essential component of a nonbacterial cell's protein-synthesis machinery. It catalyzes the transfer of adenosine diphosphate ribose, a part of the electron-carrier nicotinamide adenine dinucleotide (NAD), to a protein called elongation factor 2 (EF-2). The factor is required for the synthesis of protein on the cellular organelles called ribosomes, and it is inactivated by the attachment of the ADP-ribose group. In about a day a single diphtheria toxin molecule can inactivate most (perhaps all) of the two million EF-2 molecules in a typical animal cell. Unable to make protein, the cell dies (see Figure 12.3).

Enzymatic action of this kind, such that one toxin molecule functions repeatedly to inactivate a very large number of target molecules, is probably characteristic of most highly toxic proteins. For example, Sjur Olsnes, Alexander A. Pihl and their colleagues at Norsk Hydro's Institute for Cancer Research in Oslo have shown that ricin and some related plant toxins also depend on an enzymatic process (although it is different from diphtheria toxin's) to inactivate ribosomes.

Powerful toxins such as the ones we have described would seem to be ideal for coupling to antibodies to make an effective immunotoxin. There is a major problem, however. A toxin molecule has its own binding sites, by means of which it can bind to most mammalian cells. An immunotoxin made by simply linking a toxin molecule to an antibody retains that nonspecific binding ability. It will attach itself not only to the target cells the antibody recognizes but also to almost any other cell, and so it will kill normal cells about as efficiently as it kills cancer cells. Clearly, then, one needs somehow to eliminate the toxin's own ability to bind to cells and make it rely for binding on the antibody to which it is linked.

A way to do that emerged from detailed studies of the structure of toxic proteins done in the early 1970's. One of us (Collier), working with colleagues at the University of California at Los Angeles, and D. Michael Gill, Alwin M. Pappenheimer, Jr., and their co-workers at Harvard University found that the intact diphtheria toxin molecule would not catalyze the ADP-ribosylation of EF-2. Enzymatic activity was observed only if the toxin was first cleaved

into two unequal parts. First the long polypeptide chain of the toxin had to be cut into two smaller chains by a protease (an enzyme that attacks proteins) and then a disulfide bond linking the two chains had to be cut. (A disulfide bond is a chemical link between two sulfur atoms each of which is attached to a polypeptide chain.)

The shorter of the two resulting chains, designated the A chain, turned out to be responsible for the toxin's enzymatic activity. An A chain, separated from the longer B chain, was able to inactivate EF-2 in cell extracts. The B chain was found to be responsible for binding the toxin to receptors on the cell surface. Neither chain by itself was toxic for intact cells, implying that both binding to receptors and ADP-ribosylation are essential for the normal toxic process. Ricin and some other toxins derived from plants were found to have similar characteristics. Each such toxin is composed of two disulfide-linked chains: an A chain with enzymatic activity and a B chain serving to bind the toxin to the cell surface (see Figure 12.4).

These findings suggested to several workers that if one could couple only the A chain to a cell-specific antibody, the toxin's own receptor-binding ability should be eliminated; the antibody alone should then mediate cell-surface binding and only the target cells should be killed. Moreover, the fact that the A chain alone is virtually nontoxic (being unable to bind to cells) meant that any adventitious breakdown of the immunotoxin into A-chain and antibody components within the body would fail to yield nonspecifically toxic agents.

The fact that the two chains of the toxins we worked with are joined to each other by disulfide bonds suggested one should couple the A chain to an antibody by a similar link. Disulfide bonds are known to be ruptured easily within a cell and

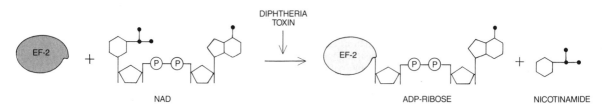

NAD   DIPHTHERIA TOXIN   ADP-RIBOSE   NICOTINAMIDE

Figure 12.3 DIPHTHERIA TOXIN acts as an enzyme. Its effect is to inactivate elongation factor 2 (EF-2), an essential component of the cell's protein-synthesizing machinery. The toxin does this by catalyzing the transfer to EF-2 of adenosine diphosphate ribose, part of the electron carrier nicotinamide adenine dinucleotide (NAD). A single molecule of diphtheria toxin can inactivate a cell's EF-2 in a single day.

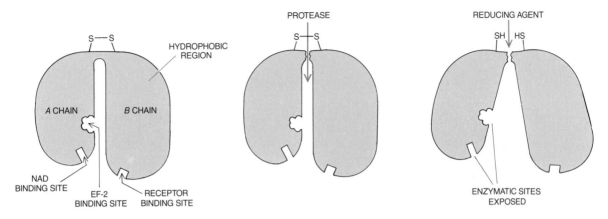

PROTEASE

REDUCING AGENT

S—S

HYDROPHOBIC REGION

A CHAIN   B CHAIN

NAD BINDING SITE

EF-2 BINDING SITE   RECEPTOR BINDING SITE

SH   HS

ENZYMATIC SITES EXPOSED

Figure 12.4 ENZYMATIC ACTIVITY is observed only after the toxin molecule (*left*) has been cleaved into two chains. The smaller one, the *A* chain, carries enzymatic sites catalyzing the transfer of ADP-ribose to EF-2. The *B* chain has a receptor-binding site and a hydrophobic region able to insert itself into a biological membrane. One way to make an immunotoxin that does not bind to nontarget cells is to use only the *A* chain. The chains are cleaved by cutting the protein bridge between them (*center*) and the disulfide bond (*S – S*) linking them (*right*).

should therefore make for easy release of the *A* chain, and thus for the chain's activation through exposure of its enzymatic site, in a target cell.

Monoclonal antibodies directed against specific cells were not then readily available, and so several groups began to test the concept by coupling *A* chains to hormones or lectins. Hormones bind to specific cell-surface receptors; the lectins, which are nontoxic plant proteins, bind avidly to various glycoproteins and glycolipids on cell surfaces. David M. Neville, Jr., and his colleagues at the National Institute of Mental Health were the first to link a toxin *A* chain to a hormone.

At UCLA, D. Gary Gilliland and one of us (Collier) linked the diphtheria toxin *A* chain to the lectin concanavalin *A*. The resulting conjugate was found to be toxic at low concentrations for human cells in culture. Its toxicity was inhibited when an excess of uncoupled concanavalin *A* was added to the culture medium. Apparently the free lectin was binding to the surface of cells, blocking the conjugate's attachment and thereby interfering with its toxic effect. This was a demonstration that the coupled lectin was indeed in control of the conjugate's binding, as we had hoped it would be. Tsuyoshi Uchida and Yoshio Okada of the University of Osaka got similar results by linking the diphtheria toxin *A* chain to a different lectin.

By the time these results had been achieved other laboratories were reporting the successful isolation of monoclonal antibodies against cell-surface antigens. Some of the antibodies were directed against tumor-associated antigens: antigens found to be present rarely, if at all, on the surface of normal cells. Zenon Steplewski and Hilary Koprowski of the Wistar Institute in Philadelphia developed a monoclonal antibody that appeared to bind to human colorectal carcinoma (CRC) cells but not to a number of other cells (see Figure 12.5). The UCLA and Wistar groups decided to collaborate to prepare immunotoxins with the anti-CRC antibody.

The immunotoxins were constructed at UCLA by linking the *A* chain of either diphtheria toxin or ricin to the antibody (see Figure 12.6). They were tested at Wistar by assaying cells for their protein-synthesizing activity, the function inhibited by the toxin. Cultured CRC cells were incubated for 24 hours with the immunotoxin, with unconjugated antibodies or *A* chains or with intact diphtheria toxin; then the cells were assayed for their ability to incorporate amino acids into proteins. Melanoma cells were tested in the same way.

The results were encouraging. Even at rather low concentrations both *A*-chain immunotoxins blocked protein synthesis effectively in the CRC cells but not in the melanoma cells, whereas the intact diphtheria toxin had a powerful effect on the melanoma cells as well as on the CRC cells. The unconjugated antibodies had no effect, and the unconjugated *A*

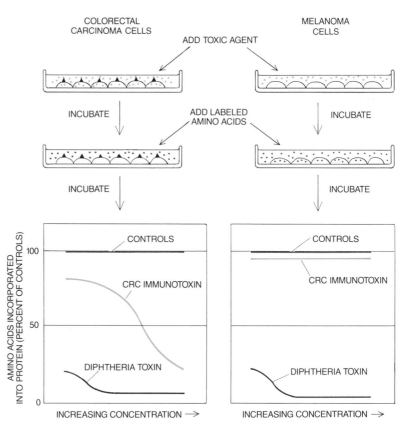

Figure 12.5 IMMUNOTOXINS made with a monoclonal antibody against colorectal carcinoma (CRC) cells were tested for their ability to inhibit protein synthesis. The immunotoxins, *A* chains or antibodies alone or intact diphtheria toxin were incubated with CRC cells and with melanoma cells. Amino acids labeled with a radioactive isotope were added and the cells' ability to incorporate them into protein was assayed. *A* chains and antibodies alone (*controls*) had little or no effect. Diphtheria toxin inhibited protein synthesis in both CRC cells (*left*) and melanoma cells (*right*). The immunotoxins were effective in CRC cells but not in melanoma cells.

chains had little effect, on either kind of cell. In other words, the antibody part of the immunotoxin did dictate specificity for CRC cells and the toxin part did have an effect on those cells. This was the first demonstration that a monoclonal antibody against a tumor-associated antigen could direct the action of a potent toxin against specific cells. At about the same time Keith A. Krolick, Ellen S. Vitetta and Jonathan W. Uhr of the University of Texas Health Science Center at Dallas reported that antibodies against a mouse leukemia-cell antigen can make the leukemia cells specific targets of the ricin A chain.

These first-generation immunotoxins made with the *A* chain alone represented only a promising initial step. Their toxicity for target cells varied widely; in some cases it was many orders of magnitude lower than that of the intact parent toxin. At about the same time as these puzzling differences in toxicity were being reported, some possible reasons for the variation were beginning to emerge. Clearly the enzymatically active part of a toxin must do its work in the cell's cytoplasm, which is where EF-2 (the diphtheria toxin's target) and the ribosomes (ricin's target) reside. Not much had been known about how a large protein gets into a cell. In our early work we hoped our lectin conjugates and then our immunotoxins would make their way to the cytoplasm, but we did not know just how that would happen, or with what efficiency.

It is now known that many proteins are brought across the cell's outer membrane, the plasma membrane, by a process called receptor-mediated endocytosis. The plasma membrane is studded with receptors, each of them specific for a particular protein or small particle. A diphtheria toxin molecule is thought to bind to such a receptor (which probably has a benign role in the ordinary life of the cell and is simply preempted by the toxin). The receptor either moves to or is already at one of many "coated pits" on the cell surface. At these

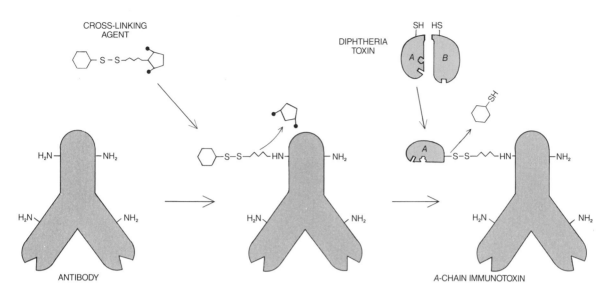

Figure 12.6 *A*-CHAIN IMMUNOTOXIN is made by conjugating an antibody against a tumor-associated antigen (*left*) with the *A* chain of diphtheria toxin. One end of a cross-linking agent carrying a disulfide bond is attached to an amino (NH$_2$) group of the antibody (*center*). The other end of the cross-linker is attached to the *A* chain of a toxin molecule (*right*); as a result the antibody replaces the toxin's *B* chain.

sites the plasma membrane invaginates, or folds inward, forming a membrane-bounded vesicle called an endosome, which carries receptors and any ligand bound to them (such as a toxin molecule) into the cell (see Figure 12.7).

A toxin molecule in an endosome is inside the cell, but it remains shielded from its substrates, EF-2 and NAD, by the endosomal membrane. How an *A* chain escapes from the endosome to get at its target has still not been clearly established. In the case of diphtheria toxin there is evidence that an increasingly acidic environment within the endosome causes the toxin molecule to insert itself into the endosomal membrane. The disulfide bond linking the *A* and *B* chains is apparently cleaved by substances called reducing compounds that are present in the cytoplasm, allowing the *A* chain to be released into the cytoplasm and leaving the *B* chain in the endosomal membrane.

Apparently, then, diphtheria toxin is an unusual, highly specialized enzyme. It must perform at least three distinct functions: binding to a receptor, insertion into and traversal of the endosomal membrane, and the transfer of ADP-ribose to EF-2. As we have explained, the first function is accomplished by the *B* chain and the last function by the *A* chain. It has recently been established that membrane insertion

is also a function of the *B* chain. It depends, in fact, on a particular region of the chain that is rich in hydrophobic amino acids, which are suited for insertion into the hydrophobic lipid membrane.

Less is known about how ricin gets into the cytoplasm. Acidity within the endosome does not seem to play a role. Nevertheless, the presence of the ricin *B* chain greatly increases the toxic activity of the ricin *A* chain, suggesting there may be a functional region of the *B* chain that (as in the case of diphtheria toxin) is operative during the *A* chain's transport into the cytoplasm.

The data on endocytosis point to two possible reasons for the reduced toxicity of *A*-chain immunotoxins compared with the toxicity of their parent toxin molecules. If, as would appear to be the case, the *A* chain can get to its substrates only by way of an endosome, the toxic activity of an immunotoxin must depend first of all on the efficiency with which it is incorporated into endosomes. That depends in turn on the ability of the cell-surface antigen to which the immunotoxin binds to transport it to a coated pit for receptor-mediated endocytosis. One reason for the reduced toxicity of certain immunotoxins may therefore be that the monoclonal antibodies with which *A* chains have been conjugated

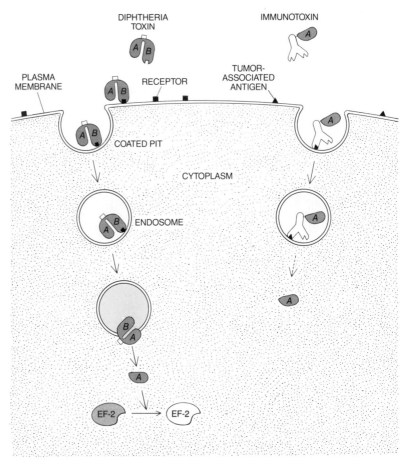

Figure 12.7 INTACT DIPHTHERIA TOXIN is thought to be taken into a cell by receptor-mediated endocytosis (*left*). The toxin's *B* chain binds to a receptor on the cell surface and the toxin is carried to one of many "coated pits," where the plasma membrane invaginates and pinches off to form an endosome. The acidic environment within the endosome (*light color*) causes the *B* chain's hydrophobic region to insert itself into the endosomal membrane; the *A* chain crosses the membrane and is released into the cytoplasm, where it inactivates EF-2. An *A*-chain immunotoxin, on the other hand, binds to a tumor-associated antigen (*right*). It may get to a coated pit and be internalized in an endosome, from which the *A* chain emerges into the cytoplasm. *A* chains reach the cytoplasm at low efficiency, however; *A*-chain immunotoxins are less effective than parent toxin molecules.

do not bind to antigens that frequent the coated pits. It should be possible, however, to find antibodies directed against such antigens.

There is a second possible reason, which may be more important. Having been carried into the cell in an endosome, the *A* chain needs to get out of the endosome to reach its substrate. At least in the case of diphtheria toxin, the membrane-insertion function required for efficient transport across the endosomal membrane is a property of the hydrophobic region of the *B* chain. By substituting an antibody for the toxin's *B* chain one therefore eliminates an activity that is critical for the efficient entry of the *A* chain into the cytoplasm. *A* chains linked to antibodies do seem to reach the cytoplasm, but they generally reach it with lower efficiency than intact toxin molecules do. Penetration of the endosomal membrane seems to be a limiting step in determining the toxic activity of an immunotoxin.

How is it possible to include in the immunotoxin the *B*-chain region required for membrane insertion without retaining the chain's receptor-binding function and thereby precluding cell-specific targeting? One approach would be to retain the entire *B* chain but block its binding to its receptors on the plasma membrane. It has long been known that the sugar lactose inhibits the binding of ricin to the surface of cells, presumably because the lactose occupies the ricin's receptor-binding site. Richard J. Youle and Neville have prepared immunotoxins by conjugating the intact ricin molecule with a monoclonal antibody. When cells in culture are treated with these whole-ricin immunotoxins in the presence of large concentrations of lactose, nonspecific toxicity is minimized. Such concentrations are toxic for animals, however, so that blocking binding sites with lactose, at least, does not appear to be feasible in human beings.

A more promising approach is to alter the *B* chain so that receptor-binding activity is eliminated but membrane-insertion activity is retained. One way to do this is to treat the intact toxin with a chemical that specifically disables only the receptor-binding part of the *B* chain and then to couple the modified toxin to an antibody. Ira H. Pastan of the National Cancer Institute and his colleagues were able to do this with *Pseudomonas* exotoxin *A*, a bacterial toxin resembling diphtheria toxin in its mode of action. No such method has yet been found for diphtheria toxin or ricin.

There is a powerful alternative way to alter the *B* chain of diphtheria toxin or ricin. Rather than modifying the toxin chemically, one can alter the gene encoding it. The new recombinant-DNA techniques make it possible to modify and manipulate genes almost it will. At UCLA we undertook the genetic engineering of toxins for the construction of immunotoxins. Our plan was to isolate the DNA coding for a toxin, to eliminate the nucleotide sequences that specify the receptor-binding site on the *B* chain and then to introduce the modified gene into *Escherichia coli* cells. The bacteria would translate the gene to make large quantities of a modified toxin: one that is unable to bind indiscriminately to cells but retains enzymatic and membrane-insertion activity, and that can be linked to a monoclonal antibody to make a cell-specific immunotoxin.

At UCLA Michael J. Bjorn and one of us (Kaplan) determined the nucleotide sequence of parts of the diphtheria-toxin gene. That enabled us to identify a fragment of the gene encoding the enzymatic and hydrophobic regions of the toxin but not the receptor-binding region. Because the protein product of the fragment would be essentially nontoxic, the Recombinant DNA Advisory Committee of the National Institutes of Health gave permission for the fragment to be cloned in *E. coli*. The fragment was cloned and then sequenced in full at the Cetus Corporation by Lawrence Greenfield, Bjorn and one of us (Kaplan). The cloned fragment is expressed in *E. coli*. The bacterial product retains the toxin's essential properties except for its ability to bind to cells.

A s for the potential medical applications of immunotoxins, perhaps the most promising one for the near future is the treatment of bone marrow in the course of transplantation. Patients with leukemia are sometimes treated by total-body irradiation or chemotherapy in an effort to kill the leuke-

mic cells. The treatment, however, also destroys normal stem cells in the bone marrow, which are the precursors of all blood cells. The patient therefore needs a bone-marrow transplant to provide a new population of stem cells. The trouble is that the transplantation can give rise to what is called graft-versus-host disease, in which *T* lymphocytes in the donated marrow recognize the recipient's cells as foreign and attack and destroy them.

To avoid this complication one would like to eliminate the *T* cells before introducing the donor's marrow into the patient. Daniel A. Vallera of the University of Minnesota Medical School and his colleagues have treated marrow cells in culture with immunotoxins made by linking intact ricin to antibodies against *T* cells. They added lactose to minimize nonspecific toxicity. The procedure reduced the marrow's *T*-cell population by about 99 percent, with minimal effect on the stem cells. The efficacy of marrow treated in this way is now being tested in patients.

Applications of this kind, in which tissues are treated by immunotoxins outside the body, are attractive as an initial step in demonstrating the effectiveness of immunotoxins. Treating cells outside the body is implicitly safer than administering the immunotoxin directly to a patient, because one can remove any excess immunotoxin by rinsing the cells before injecting them into the recipient.

The long-term challenge, however, is to develop immunotoxins into a new family of chemotherapeutic agents with which to treat patients directly. Tests of immunotoxins have been done in animals, with some reports of tumor regression, or reduction in size. For example, Michael I. Bernhard of the National Cancer Institute and his colleagues treated liver carcinoma in guinea pigs with an immunotoxin consisting of the diphtheria toxin *A* chain linked by a disulfide bond to a monoclonal antibody directed against an antigen on the cancer cells. A single dose of the immunotoxin led to tumor regression but did not completely eradicate the tumor.

M uch research still needs to be done; on antibodies, on toxic agents and on methods of treatment. Many laboratories are now at work isolating monoclonal antibodies against various human cancers. Almost certainly a large number of different immunotoxins will have to be developed whose antibody portions are specific for various tumor-associated antigens on different cancer cells. As we mentioned above, a radioactive isotope or one of the conventional chemotherapeutic agents could be coupled to these antibodies instead of a modified natural toxin. It is also possible that antibodies will be found that by themselves can initiate an attack by the patient's own immune system against cancer cells.

It is likely that genetic engineering will play an increasing role in the development of immunotoxins. Just as one can eliminate the receptor-binding region of the B chain by manipulating the diphtheria toxin gene, so one can modify toxin genes in other ways to improve the efficacy and safety of toxin molecules. Eventually it may be possible to make the entire immunotoxin by genetic-engineering techniques: to isolate the gene for a wanted monoclonal antibody, perhaps modify it to improve its affinity for a particular antigen, link it to an appropriate toxin gene and let bacteria or such eukaryotic cells as yeasts synthesize the immunotoxin as a single construct.

In the human body an immunotoxin will be subjected to an environment much more complex than that of a cell culture. To be effective an immunotoxin must remain stable as it moves through the circulatory system, must be able to gain access to target cells in many parts of the body and of course must not damage normal tissues that are crucial to survival. The degree to which various immunotoxins satisfy these requirements is currently under study. The task of alleviating or curing cancer by chemotherapy is a formidable one. Probably no single approach will suffice. Immunotoxins may become one of many weapons in the armamentarium.

The Authors

The Editor

WILLIAM E. PAUL is chief of the Laboratory of Immunology of the National Institute of Allergy and Infectious Diseases (NIAID) at the National Institutes of Health. He received his M.D. from the State University of New York, Downstate Medical Center in 1960 and, after clinical training at Massachusetts Memorial Hospital in Boston, was a clinical associate at the National Cancer Institute and then a post-doctoral fellow at New York University School of Medicine. He joined NIAID in 1968 and assumed his present position in 1970.

GORDON L. ADA and **SIR GUSTAV NOSSAL** ("The Clonal-Selection Theory") worked together on studies that helped to establish the theory they recount. Ada is professor of microbiology at the Johns Hopkins School of Public Health. His undergraduate and graduate degrees are from the University of Sydney, where he received his Ph.D. in 1959. From 1946 to 1948 he was at the National Institute for Medical Research in London. He then joined the staff of the Walter and Eliza Hall Institute of Medical Research in Melbourne, leaving in 1968 for the Curtin School. Nossal has been director of the Hall Institute and professor of medical biology at the University of Melbourne since 1965. He studied medicine at the University of Sydney and in 1960 received his Ph.D. from Melbourne. After two years as assistant professor of genetics at the Stanford University School of Medicine, Nossal went to the Hall Institute as deputy director. He has also been a visiting scientist at the Pasteur Institute in Paris and a consultant to the World Health Organization.

PHILIP LEDER ("The Genetics of Antibody Diversity") is John Emory Andrus Professor of Genetics and chairman of the department of genetics at the Harvard Medical School. He received his bachelor's degree in 1956 from Harvard College and his M.D. in 1960 from the Harvard Medical School. In 1962 he went to the National Heart Institute as a research associate, then served as a research medical officer of the National Cancer Institute, head of the section on molecular genetics of the National Institute of Child Health and

Human Development and chief of the laboratory of molecular genetics of the NICHD. He moved to Harvard in 1980.

PHILIPPA MARRACK and **JOHN KAPPLER** ("The T Cell and Its Receptor") are a wife-and-husband team at the National Jewish Center for Immunology and Respiratory Medicine in Denver. Both are professors of medicine at the University of Colorado Health Sciences Center, where Marrack is also professor of biochemistry, biophysics and genetics and Kappler is also professor of microbiology and immunology. Marrack received her undergraduate training and Ph.D. (1970) at the University of Cambridge. Kappler received his undergraduate degree at Lehigh University in 1965 and his Ph.D. from Brandeis University in 1970. The two investigators were postdoctoral fellows together at the University of California at San Diego before going to the University of Rochester Medical School in 1973 and Colorado in 1979.

HOWARD M. GREY, ALESSANDRO SETTE and **SØREN BUUS** ("How T Cells See Antigen") have been long-time collaborators in the study of antigen processing and presentation. Grey is cofounder and chief technical officer of the Cytel Corporation in La Jolla, Calif., a biotechnology company that is designing immune-modulating drugs. He received his M.D. from New York University in 1957 and has done research at the Scripps Clinic and Research Foundation and at the National Jewish Center for Immunology and Respiratory Medicine. Sette is senior staff scientist at Cytel and assistant professor of immunology at Scripps. He received his Ph.D. from the University of Rome in 1984 and joined Grey at the National Jewish Center in 1986. Buus, who earned an M.D. at the University of Aarhus in 1981, is assistant professor at the Institute of Experimental Immunology at the University of Copenhagen.

KENDALL A. SMITH ("Interleukin-2) is professor of medicine at Dartmouth Medical School. He received his M.D. from Ohio State University College of Medicine in 1968. After completing his clinical medical training at Yale University, he devoted several years to postdoctoral research at the National Cancer Institute, Dartmouth and the Institute for Cancer Research and Immunogenetics in Villejuif, France.

LLOYD J. OLD ("Tumor Necrosis Factor") holds the William E. Snee Chair of Cancer Immunology at the Memorial Sloan-Kettering Cancer Center in New York, where he has worked since he received his M.D. at the University of California School of Medicine in 1958. From 1973 to 1983 he served as vice-president and associate director of scientific development at the Sloan-Kettering Institute for Cancer Research. He is also scientific director of the Ludwig Institute for Cancer Research.

JOHN DING-E YOUNG and ZANVIL A. COHN ("How Killer Cells Kill") work together in the Cohn/Steinman laboratory of cellular physiology and immunology at Rockefeller University. Young, an assistant professor at Rockefeller, obtained an M.D. in 1979 at the National University of Brasilia and then completed his Ph.D. and a two-year fellowship at Rockefeller before assuming his current position in 1985. Cohn is professor and senior physician at Rockefeller and adjunct professor of medicine at the Cornell University Medical College. He received his M.D. at the Harvard Medical School in 1953 and did his internship and residency at the Massachusetts General Hospital. After serving as chief of the division of rickettsial biology at the Walter Reed Army Institute, he went to Rockefeller in 1958.

IRUN R. COHEN ("The Self, the World and Autoimmunity") is Mauerberger Professor of Immunology at the Weizmann Institute of Science in Israel. He received his M.D. at Northwestern University. After doing an internship and spending two years at the Communicable Disease Center in Atlanta, he completed a residency in pediatrics at the Johns Hopkins Hospital. He moved in 1968 to the Weizmann Institute, where he has been ever since, except for a period

in the early 1970's when he helped to establish a medical school at the Ben-Gurion University in Beer-Sheva.

STEVEN A. ROSENBERG ("Adoptive Immunotherapy for Cancer") has been chief of surgery at the National Cancer Institute since 1974. He earned his M.D. from the Johns Hopkins University School of Medicine in 1963 and his Ph.D. in biophysics from Harvard University in 1968. He completed a surgical residency at the Peter Bent Brigham Hospital in Boston before accepting his current post.

CESAR MILSTEIN ("Monoclonal Antibodies") is a senior member of the British Medical Research Council Laboratory of Molecular Biology in Cambridge. He graduated from the University of Buenos Aires in 1952 with a degree in chemical sciences and received his Ph.D. in 1957 from the university's Institute of Biological Chemistry. In 1958 he joined the department of biochemistry at the University of Cambridge, where he received a Ph.D. in 1960. After heading the division of molecular biology at the National Microbiological Institute in Buenos Aires, Milstein returned to Cambridge. Milstein and his colleagues received a Nobel Prize in 1984 for their work in immunology.

RICHARD A. LERNER and ALFONSO TRAMONTANO ("Catalytic Antibodies") are at the Research Institute of Scripps Clinic: Lerner is director of the institute and Tramontano is an associate member in the department of molecular biology. Lerner received his M.D. in 1964 at the Stanford University School of Medicine and has been at Scripps since 1965, except for two years at the Wistar Institute of Anatomy and Biology in Philadelphia. Tramontano received a bachelor's degree in 1976 at Columbia University and a Ph.D. in inorganic chemistry from the University of California at Riverside in 1980. He went to Scripps in 1983 after he completed postdoctoral studies at Harvard University.

R. JOHN COLLIER and DONALD A. KAPLAN ("Immunotoxins") are respectively a professor of microbiology at the Harvard Medical School and a molecular geneticist at the Dow Chemical Company. Collier received a B.A. from Rice University and his Ph.D. in biology from Harvard University. Kaplan received a B.A. and his Ph.D. in biology from UCLA. After serving as research molecular geneticist in the department of microbiology at UCLA he became senior scientist and project manager of immunotoxins at Cetus in 1981. He left Cetus in 1984 to become senior associate scientist at Dow.

Bibliographies

1. The Clonal-Selection Theory

Ehrlich, Paul. 1900. Croonian lecture. On immunity with special reference to cell life. *Proceedings of the Royal Society of London* 66 (July 24): 424–448.

Jerne, Niels K. 1955. The natural-selection theory of antibody formation. *Proceedings of the National Academy of Sciences* 41 (November): 849–857.

Burnet, F. M. 1957. A modification of Jerne's theory of antibody production using the concept of clonal selection. *The Australian Journal of Science* 20 (October 21): 67–69.

Talmage, David W. 1986. The acceptance and rejection of immunological concepts. *Annual Review of Immunology* 4:1–11.

2. The Genetics of Antibody Diversity

Dreyer, W. J., and J. Claude Bennett. 1965. The molecular basis of antibody formation: A paradox. *Proceedings of the National Academy of Sciences* 54 (September): 864–868.

Hozumi, Nobumichi, and Susumu Tonegawa. 1976. Evidence for somatic rearrangement of immunoglobulin genes coding for variable and constant regions. *Proceedings of the National Academy of Sciences* 73 (October): 3628–3632.

Max, Edward E., J. G. Seidman and Philip Leder. 1979. Sequences of five potential recombination sites encoded close to an immunoglobulin κ constant region gene. *Proceedings of the National Academy of Sciences* 76 (July): 3450–3454.

Leder, Philip, Edward E. Max and J. G. Seidman. 1980. The organization of immunoglobulin genes and the origin of their diversity. In *Immunology 80*, eds. M. Fougereau and J. Dausset. Academic Press.

3. The T Cell and Its Receptor

Zinkernagel, Rolf M., and Peter C. Doherty. 1975. *H-2* compatibility requirement for *T*-cell mediated lysis of target cells infected with lymphocytic choriomeningitis virus: Different cytotoxic *T*-cell specificities are associated with structures coded from *H2K* or *H-2D*. *The Journal of Experimental Medicine* 141 (June 1): 1427–1436.

Kappler, John W., Barry Skidmore, Janice White and Philippa Marrack. 1981. Antigen-inducible, *H-2*-restricted, interleukin-2-producing *T* cell hybridomas lack of independent antigen and *H-2* recognition. *The Journal of Experimental Medicine* 153 (May 1): 1198–1214.

Babbitt, Bruce P., Paul M. Allen, Gary Matsueda, Edgar Haber and Emil R. Unanue. 1985. Binding of immunogenic peptides to Ia histocompatability molecules. *Nature* 317 (September 26): 359–361.

4. How T Cells See Antigen

Unanue, Emil R. 1984. Antigen presenting function of the macrophage. *Annual Review of Immunology* 2:395–428.

Braciale, Thomas J., et al. 1987. Antigen presentation pathways to class I and class II MHC-restricted *T* lymphocytes. *Immunological Reviews* (August): 95–114.

Buus, Søren, Alessandro Sette and Howard M. Grey. 1987. The interaction between protein-derived immunogenic peptides and Ia. *Immunological Reviews* (August): 115–141.

Bjorkman, P. J., et al. 1987. Structure of the human class I histocompatibility antigen, HLA-A2. *Nature* 329 (October 8): 506–512.

5. Interleukin-2

Burnet, Sir Macfarlane. 1969. *Cellular immunology.* Melbourne University Press.

Smith, Kendall A., ed. 1988. *Interleukin 2.* Academic Press.

Smith, Kendall A., ed. 1988. *Interleukin-2.* Inception, impact, and implications. *Science* 240 (May 27): 1169–1176.

———. 1989. The interleukin 2 receptor. In *Annual Review of Cell Biology*, vol. 5, ed. G. E. Palade.

6. Tumor Necrosis Factor

Oppenheim, Joost J., David L. Rosenstreich and Michael Potter, eds. 1981. *Cellular functions in immunity and inflammation.* Elsevier North-Holland, Inc.

Old, Lloyd J. 1985. Tumor necrosis factor (TNF). *Science* 230 (November 8): 630–632.

Bock, Gregory, and Joan Marsh, eds. 1987. *Tumor necrosis factor and related cytotoxins.* John Wiley & Sons, Inc.

Nathan, Carl F. 1987. Secretory products of macrophages. *Journal of Clinical Investigation* 79 (February): 319–326.

Bonavida, Benjamin, George E. Gifford, Holger Kirchner and Lloyd J. Old, eds. 1988. *Tumor necrosis factor/cachectin and related cytokines.* S. Karger, AG, Basel.

7. How Killer Cells Kill

Henkart, Pierre A. 1985. Mechanism of lymphocyte-mediated cytotoxicity. *Annual Review of Immunology* 3:31–58.

Podack, Eckhard R. 1985. Molecular mechanism of lymphocyte mediated tumor lysis. *Immunology Today* 6:21–27.

Young, John Ding-E, Hans Hengartner, Eckhard R. Podack and Zanvil A. Cohn. 1986. Purification and characterization of a cytolytic pore-forming protein from granules of cloned lymphocytes with natural killer activity. *Cell* 44 (March 28): 849–859.

Young, John Ding-E, William R. Clark, Chau-Ching Liu and Zanvil A. Cohn. 1987. A calcium- and perforin-independent pathway of killing mediated by murine cytolytic lymphocytes. *The Journal of Experimental Medicine* 166 (December): 1894–1899.

8. The Self, the World and Autoimmunity

Holoshitz, Joseph, Yaakov Naparstek, Avraham Ben-Nun and Irun R. Cohen. 1983. Lines of *T* lymphocytes induce or vaccinate against autoimmune arthritis. *Science* 219 (January 7): 56–58.

Cohen, Irun R., Dana Elias, Ruth Maron and Yoram Schechter. 1984. Immunization to insulin generates antidiotypes that behave as antibodies to the insulin hormone receptor and cause diabetes mellitus. In *Idiotypy in Biology and Medicine*, eds. Heinz Köhler, Jacques Urbain and Pierre-André Cazenave. Academic Press, Inc.

Cohen, Irun R., Joseph Holoshitz, Willem van Eden and Ayalla Frenkel. 1985. *T* lymphocyte clones illuminate pathogenesis and affect therapy of experimental arthritis. *Arthritis and Rheumatism* 28 (August): 841–845.

Van Eden, Willem, Jelle E. R. Thole, Ruurd van der Zee, Alie Noordzij, Jan D. A. van Embden, Evert J. Hensen and Irun R. Cohen. 1988. Cloning of the mycobacterial epitope recognized by *T* lymphocytes in adjuvant arthritis. *Nature* 331 (January 14): 171–173.

9. Adoptive Immunotherapy for Cancer

DeVita, Vincent T., Jr., Samuel Hellman and Steven A. Rosenberg, eds. 1986. *Important advances in oncology.* J. B. Lippincott Co.

Rosenberg, Steven A. 1988. The development of new immunotherapies for the treatment of cancer using interleukin-2. *Annals of Surgery* 208 (August): 121–135.

Rosenberg, S. A., B. S. Packard, P. M. Aebersold, D. Solomon, S. L. Topalian, S. T. Toy, P. Simon, M. T. Lotze, J. C. Yang, C. A. Seipp, C. Simpson, C. Carter, S. Bock, D. Schwartzentruber, J. P. Wei and D. E. White. 1988. Use of tumor-infiltrating lymphocytes and interleukin-2 in the immunotherapy of patients with metastatic melanoma: A preliminary report. *New England Journal of Medicine* 319 (December 22): 1676–1680.

Rosenberg, S. A., M. T. Lotze, J. C. Yang, P. M. Aebersold, W. M. Linehan, C. A. Seipp and D. E. White. 1989. Experience with the use of high-dose interleukin-2 in the treatment of 652 cancer patients. *Annals of Surgery* 210 (October): 474–485.

10. Monoclonal Antibodies

Köhler, G., and C. Milstein. 1976. Derivation of specific antibody-producing tissue culture and tumor lines by cell fusion. *European Journal of Immunology* 6:511–519.

Melchers, F., Basel M. Potter and N. Warner, eds. 1978. Lymphocyte hybridomas. *Current Topics in Microbiology and Immunology.* Springer-Verlag.

Möller, Göran, ed. 1979. Hybrid myeloma monoclonal antibodies against MHC products. *Immunological Reviews* 47:3–252.

Milstein, C., G. Galfre, D. S. Secher and T. Spring. 1979. Monoclonal antibodies and cell surface antigens. *Ciba Foundation Symposia*, no. 66: 251–276.

11. Catalytic Antibodies

Lienhard, Gustav E. 1973. Enzymatic catalysis and transition-state theory. *Science* 180 (April 13): 149–154.

Gandour, Richard D., and Richard L. Schowen, eds. 1978. *Transition states in biochemical processes.* Plenum Press.

Fersht, Alan. 1985. *Enzyme structure and mechanism.* W. H. Freeman and Company.

Tramontano, Alfonso, Kim D. Janda and Richard A. Lerner. 1986. Catalytic antibodies. *Science* 234 (December 19): 1566–1570.

Napper, Andrew D., Stephen J. Benkovic, Alfonso Tramontano and Richard A. Lerner. 1987. A stereospecific cyclization catalyzed by an antibody. *Science* 237 (August 28): 1041–1043.

12. Immunotoxins

Gilliland, D. Gary, Zenon Steplewski, R. John Collier, Kenneth F. Mitchell, Tony H. Chang and Hilary Koprowski. 1980. Antibody-directed cytotoxic agents: Use of monoclonal antibody to direct the action of toxin *A* chains to colrectal carcinoma cells. *Proceedings of the National Academy of Sciences* 77 (August): 4539–4543.

———. 1982. Antibody carriers of drugs and toxins in tumor therapy. *Immunological Reviews* 62:5–216.

Olsnes, Sjur, and Alexander Pihl. 1982. Chimeric toxins. *Pharmacology and Therapeutics* 15:355–381.

Greenfield, Lawrence, Michael J. Bjorn, Glenn Horn, Darlene Fong, Gregory A. Buck, R. John Collier and Donald A. Kaplan. 1983. Nucleotide sequence of the structural gene for diphtheria toxin carried by corynebacteriophage *β*. *Proceedings of the National Academy of Sciences* 80 (November): 6853–6857.

Sources of the Photographs

James G. Hirsch: Figure 1.1

Walter and Eliza Hall Institute of Medical Research: Figure 1.5 (*top and bottom*)

David W. Talmage, University of Colorado School of Medicine: Figure 1.5 (*right*)

Richard J. Feldman, National Institute of Health: Figure 2.1

Morton H. Nielsen and Ole Werdelin, University of Copenhagen: Figure 4.1

Mark A. Saper, Harvard University: Figure 4.5 (*top*)

Helen Coley Nauts, Cancer Research Institute: Figure 6.1

Lloyd J. Old: Figures 6.2 and 6.3

Michael A. Gimbrone, Jr., Harvard Medical School: Figure 6.5

Edward A. Havell and Robert J. North, Trudeau Institute, Inc.: Figure 6.7

Barbara D. Williamson, Memorial Sloan-Kettering Cancer Center: Figure 6.8

Gilla Kaplan, Rockefeller University: Figures 7.1 and 7.7

John Ding-E Young, Rockefeller University: Figures 7.2 and 7.3

Ritta Stanescu, Hôpital des Enfants Malades, Paris: Figure 8.2

Steven A. Rosenberg: Figures 9.2 and 9.5 (*bottom*)

Cesar Milstein and Georges Köhler: Figure 10.2

Elizabeth D. Getzoff and John A. Tainer: Figure 11.1

Michael E. Pique, Elizabeth D. Getzoff and John A. Tainer: Figure 11.2

Arthur J. Olson: Figure 11.6

Arthur E. Frankel, Cetus Corporation: Figure 12.1

INDEX

Page numbers in *italics* indicate illustrations.